THE COOKBOOK THAT TELLS YOU HOW

The Retirement Food and Nutrition Manual

Brother Herman E. Zaccarelli, C. S. C.

Volume I

Published for and distributed by
United Societies of U.S.A.
Scranton Life Building
Scranton, Pennsylvania 18503
(717) 342–3294

Cahners Books
A Division of Cahners Publishing Company, Inc.
89 Franklin Street
Boston, Massachusetts 02110

Library of Congress Catalog Card Number: 75-6894
ISBN: 0-8436-2078-1

Printed in the United States of America

This book is dedicated to Thomas A. Ryan, former general manager of the L. J. Minor Corporation, Cleveland, Ohio.

By his charisma, his beauty, his charm, his sensitivity and love, he inspired the author to develop this book as a service to the 21 million Americans of all ethnic groups who are living on retirement incomes.

Great chefs of the world hold him in high esteem. He has done more for the development and appreciation of fine cuisine in America than anyone else before or after him. He appreciated and loved life and was a living example that the golden years can be creative years with food. He had the wisdom to enjoy to the fullest the seasons of life.

There is a season for everything
and a time for every purpose under heaven

A time to be born
and a time to die

A time to plant
and a time to reap

A time to hurt
and a time to heal

A time to tear down
and a time to build up

A time to cry
and a time to laugh

A time to cast away stones
and a time to gather stones together

A time to embrace
and a time to refrain from embracing

A time to gain
and a time to lose

A time to keep
and a time to throw away

A time to rend
and a time to sow

A time to speak
and a time to be silent

A time to love
and a time to hate

A time for war
and a time for peace

What has a man to show for his trying?
What is the meaning of it all?

Ecclesiastes 3: 1–11

Contents

Introduction

The Cookbook That Tells You How was conceived by the United Societies of U.S.A., a nonprofit fraternal organization, as a public service to the 21 million Americans living on retirement incomes and the millions of persons of all ages on restricted diets.

This manual, the first of its kind, features all the information needed to eat well despite inflation and despite dietary restrictions.

We have developed unique checklist chapters on purchasing and food preparation. This will enable a person to become a more critical shopper. It will also present, in simple, direct style, the art of food preparation and the utilization of leftover foods to contribute to better maintenance of our mental and physical well-being.

A special feature of the book is 1,095 menus plus special menus for holidays.

Special diets have been given priority. In addition to regular diets, we have included special recipes and diets for those who are diabetic. Other restricted diets include sodium restricted diets, low fat diets, liquid diets, high carbohydrate diets, high protein and special allergy diets.

This book is intended to bring joy and creativity into your lives through festive meals that are economical and thrifty.

Food Purchasing Checklist

Purchasing food is an art as well as a science. The art is simple, and the science is not difficult if you follow a list of minimum rules. If you do, you will enjoy savings and economy, while enjoying the maximum quality of foods.

GENERAL RECOMMENDATIONS

Plan your menus one week in advance according to the basic menu plan in the menu planning chapter. This system will enable you to utilize the unused foods that you already have on hand.

Prepare a shopping list, grouping items by the order you find them in the supermarket.

Plan at least one-third to one-half of your weekly menus around the weekly advertising specials.

Become familiar with brand names so that you will be able to recognize price changes. A price increase in one will tell you to compare brands and to switch to the lower priced brands.

Learn to read labels carefully to find the best buy nutritionally and costwise.

Learn to compare costs for the same food in the fresh, frozen, and canned sections of your supermarket.

Learn to purchase by weight rather than by volume, package size, or number.

Shop after you have had your meal. If you go to the store hungry, your shopping list will increase considerably.

Never economize on nutrition. Shop for foods that are good sources of important nutrients, and buy as many of these foods as your budget allows, with the greatest possible variety of foods you enjoy.

Shop competitively, perhaps at two or three supermarkets to take advantage of the sales in each, if the supermarkets are close together.

All chain supermarkets have their own brands. Purchase these products instead of name brands—it almost always results in savings. A general range of products to be found under the supermarket brands are canned and frozen vegetables and fruits, sandwich spreads, oils and shortenings, paper products, tea, coffee, soft drinks, and laundry products. Store brand margarine, for example, is usually lower in price than shortening. Store brand flour usually has no coupons or recipes, but it is enriched and lower in price than others.

MEATS

Beef

Beef varies in quality more than any other kind of meat. The United States Department of Agriculture grades are the most reliable guide to meat quality.

U.S.D.A. Prime. Prime grade beef is the ultimate in tenderness, juiciness, and flavor. It has abundant marbling—flecks of fat with the lean—which enhances both flavor and juices. Unless it is a very special occasion, this grade of beef should not be used.

U.S.D.A. Choice. This grade of beef often pleases thrifty shoppers because it is somewhat leaner than the higher grade. It is relatively tender, but because it has less marbling, it lacks some of the juiciness and flavor of the higher grade.

U.S.D.A. Standard. Standard grade of beef has a high portion of lean meat and little fat. Because it comes from young animals, beef of this grade is fairly tender. Because it lacks marbling, it is very mild in flavor and most cuts will be somewhat dry unless prepared by moist heat.

U.S.D.A. Commercial. Commercial grade is produced only from mature animals—the top three grades are restricted to young animals. It does not have abundant marbling (compare it with the Prime grade) and will require long, slow cooking with moist heat to make it tender.

Lamb

There are two grades of lamb that are used the most in today's market.

U.S.D.A. Prime. Prime grade lamb is very tender, juicy,

and flavorful. It has generous marbling, which enhances both flavor and juiciness. Prime chops and roasts are excellent for dry heat cooking—broiling and roasting. However, for economy, we suggest U.S.D.A. Choice.

U.S.D.A. Choice. Choice grade lamb has slightly less marbling than Prime, but still is of very high quality. Like Prime, chops and roasts are very tender, juicy, and flavorful and are suited to dry heat cooking.

Pork

Pork is the least used meat among the elderly. Like lamb, pork is generally produced from young animals and is therefore less variable in quality than beef. The U.S. Department of Agriculture grades for pork reflect only two levels of quality—acceptable and unacceptable. Unacceptable quality pork, which includes that having meat that is soft and watery, is graded U.S. Utility. All higher grades must have an acceptable quality of lean meat. The differences between these higher grades are numerical, ranging from U.S. Number 1 to U.S. Number 4, and are solely those of the yield of the four major lean cuts. In this respect, they are similar to yield grades for beef and lamb. In general, grades are not identified by the consumer at the retail level.

In purchasing pork, look for cuts with a relatively small amount of fat over the outside and with meat that is firm and a grayish pink color. For the most delicious taste, the meat should have a small amount of marbling.

POULTRY

Select by Grade

When grading is done in cooperation with the state, the official grade shield may include the words "Federal State Graded."

U.S. Grade A. The highest quality is U.S. Grade A. Grade A birds are fully fleshed and meaty, well finished, and attractive in appearance.

U.S. Grade B. Grade B birds may be less attractive in finish and appearance and slightly lacking in meatiness. Grade B is seldom printed on poultry labels.

Select by Class

The grade of poultry does not indicate how tender the bird is—the age (class) of the bird is the determining factor. Young birds are more tender than older ones. Young, tender-meated classes are most suitable for barbecuing, frying, broiling, or roasting. Mature, less tender-meated classes may be preferred for stewing, baking, soups, or salads. Mature turkeys may be labeled mature turkey, yearling turkey, or old turkey.

EGGS

Select by Grade

Grade refers to interior quality and the condition of the shell. The U.S.D.A. has listed the following grades.

Grade AA. Egg covers small area; white is thick, stands high; yolk is firm and high.

Grade A. Egg covers moderate area; white is thick, stands high; yolk is firm and high.

These higher quality eggs are ideal for all purposes, but are especially good for frying and poaching where appearance is important.

Grade B. These eggs are good for general cooking and baking, where appearance is not important.

Select by Size

The size refers to minimum weight per dozen. The size is shown within the grade seal or elsewhere on the carton. Size and quality are not related; they are entirely different. For example, large eggs may be of high or low quality; high quality eggs may be either large or small.

Egg prices vary by size for the same grade. The amount of price variation depends on the supply of the various sizes. Usually there is a 7 cent price range between one size and the next smaller size in the same grade. You will, of course, secure more for your money by purchasing the larger size.

Color

Shell color is determined by the breed of the hen and does not affect the grade, nutritive value, flavor, or cooking performance of the egg.

CANNED VEGETABLES

Canned vegetables provide many of the vitamins, minerals and food energy we need as part of our daily diet. All canned vegetables are wholesome and nutritious, but they do differ in quality. The difference in quality means a difference in the taste, texture, and appearance of the vegetable and also in its price. The grades point out the difference.

Select by Grade

U.S. Grade standards—measures of quality—have been established for most processed vegetables by the U.S. Department of Agriculture's Consumer and Marketing Service.

U.S. Grade A or Fancy. Grade A vegetables are carefully selected for color, tenderness, and lack of blemishes. They are the most tender, succulent, and flavorful vegetables produced.

U.S. Grade B or Extra Standard. Grade B or Extra Standard vegetables are of excellent quality but not quite so well selected for color and tenderness as Grade A. They are usually slightly more mature and, therefore, they have a slightly different taste than the more succulent vegetables in Grade A.

U.S. Grade C or Standard. Grade C vegetables are not so uniform in color and flavor as vegetables in the higher grades, and they are usually mature. They are a thrifty buy when appearance is not too important—for instance, when you are using them as an ingredient in a soup or soufflé.

The grade you purchase depends on your taste and your budget. Grade A or Fancy vegetables in whole or fancy cut styles are probably the most expensive vegetables, but they are the most tender and flavorful and they make the most attractive servings.

Grade B or Extra Standard vegetables are less expensive. They are delicious served hot or in casseroles or gelatin salads.

Grade C or Standard vegetables are usually diced and in pieces. They are also less expensive and are used in soups, purees, or soufflés.

All three grades, in any style, are wholesome and nutritious.

When purchasing canned vegetables, be sure that the cans are not leaking or swelled or bulged at either end. Bulging or swelling indicates spoilage. Small dents in the can do not harm the contents.

Vegetables sold in glass jars with screw and vacuum sealed lids are sealed tightly to preserve the contents. If there is any indication that the lid has been tampered with, return the jar to the supermarket and report the matter to the manager.

CANNED FRUITS

Canned fruits preserved at the peak of goodness are ready to serve as they come from the container. They are convenient to use and are always available.

Processed fruits differ in quality, taste, texture, and appearance and are usually priced according to their quality. Different qualities of fruits are suited to different uses. You can secure better buys by choosing processed fruits in the quality that fits your personal needs.

Select by Grade

U.S. Grade standards—measures of quality—have been established for most processed fruits by the U.S. Department of Agriculture's Consumer and Marketing Service.

U.S. Grade A or Fancy. Grade A fruits are the very best, with an excellent color and uniform size, weight, and shape. Having the proper ripeness and few or no blemishes, fruits of this grade are excellent to use for special purposes where appearance and flavor are important.

U.S. Grade B or Choice. Grade B fruits make up many of the fruits that are processed and are of very good quality. Only slightly less perfect than Grade A in color, uniformity, and texture, Grade B fruits have good flavor and are suitable for most uses.

U.S. Grade C or Standard. Grade C fruits may contain some broken and uneven pieces. Although flavor may not be as sweet as in higher qualities, these fruits are still good and wholesome. They are most useful where color and texture are not of great importance, such as in puddings, jams, and frozen desserts.

Read the Labels

Federal regulations require that the following information be included on the front panel of the label of a can.

1. The common or usual name of the fruit.

2. The form or style of fruit, such as whole, slices, or halves.

3. For some fruits, the variety of color.

4. Syrups, sugar, or liquid in which a fruit is packed must be listed near the name of the product.

5. The total contents (net weight) must be stated in ounces for containers holding one pound or less. From one to four pounds, weight must be given in both total ounces and pounds.

FRESH VEGETABLES

The U.S. Department of Agriculture has established two or more grades for fresh vegetables. The top grades in most cases are U.S. Number 1 or U.S. Fancy. These standards are used as a basis for trading between growers, shippers, wholesalers, and retailers. The quality of most fresh vegetables can be judged by their external appearance. Sharp-eyed consumers like yourself can make good selections of fresh vegetables from retail display counters, even though they may not bear marks or other identification of quality at this stage of sale.

Do not purchase fresh vegetables just because of a low price. It seldom pays to purchase fresh vegetables merely because the price is low. Unless the lower price is a result of overabundance of the vegetable at the time, the so-called bargain may be undesirable.

Purchase only what you need for the week—even if the product is a good buy, since some fresh vegetables deteriorate rapidly.

Purchase fresh vegetables in season, since quality is usually higher and prices more reasonable when you purchase in season. Out of season produce is generally more expensive.

Purchase the plentiful foods. The U.S. Department of

Agriculture tells you each month which vegetables are in the greatest supply and worthy of your special attention. These foods are reasonably priced.

FRESH FRUITS

Check the characteristic signs of freshness such as bright, lively color and crispness. Fruits are usually at their best quality and price at the peak of the season.

Use thoughtful care to prevent injury to fruit. Some fruits are hardier than others, but bruising and damage can be prevented by just being careful. The consumer pays for carelessness in the long run.

The U.S. Department of Agriculture notifies consumers through newspapers and other media when fruits are in abundant supply across the country. Shop for the fruits that are plentiful.

Do not purchase fruits just because of a low price. It is not to your advantage to purchase more fresh fruits than you can properly store in your refrigerator or than you can use without waste. Most fresh fruit can be stored for 10 days.

Do not purchase fresh fruit affected by decay. Even if you do trim off the decayed area, rapid deterioration is likely to spread to the salvaged area. To pay a few cents extra for fresh fruits in good condition is a good investment.

CONVENIENCE FOODS

Select a minimum of built-in convenience foods.

Make selections from your frozen food section last, and put them in your freezer as soon as you return home. Frozen foods stay in prime condition longer if they are not subject to drastic temperature changes and if your freezer is set at $0°$ or below.

Frozen potatoes may often be cheaper than fresh ones, and they offer a time saving, too. They can be fried or boiled for use in potato salad, for example.

Instant nonfat dry milk can be whipped if mixed with equal parts of lukewarm water or fruit juice, and it is much less expensive than whipped cream.

Food Preparation Checklist

The preparation of food is an art as well as a science. The art is simple, and the science becomes easy and enjoyable if we observe simple rules. This food preparation checklist will assist you in becoming the cook who will be a master-creator, savoring the many joys of food preparation.

MEATS

How to Roast Meat

1. Rub the roast with salt and pepper, other seasonings if you wish.
2. Place it, fat side up, on a rack in a shallow roasting pan.
3. Stick your meat thermometer into the meat so that its tip is in the center of the thickest muscle, resting in meat, not on bone or in fat.
4. Slide the pan into a 325° oven and forget it until along toward the end of your estimated cooking time. No basting, no water in the pan, no cover.

How to Braise Meat

1. Season meat and dip it in flour, if you like, or if you have pork chops or veal cutlets, coat with egg and crumbs if you wish.
2. Brown evenly in a small amount of fat in a heavy skillet or pot. In the case of uncoated pork chops, the pork fat is sufficient for browning.
3. Cover and cook slowly on top of the range or in the oven at 325°, until meat is tender when pierced with a fork. A small amount of liquid—water, wine, tomato juice, cream or canned soup—may be added.

How to Broil Meat

1. Place meat on broiler rack 3 to 5 inches from preheated (500–550°) broiler unit. Thick steaks and frozen ones should be farthest from the heat.
2. Broil until brown on one side. Season with salt and pepper (except ham).
3. Turn and brown second side. Season with salt and pepper.
4. Serve at once with pan drippings.

How to Fry Meats

Thin pieces of tender meat and leftover cooked meats may be fried or French fried. Chops may be floured or breaded (dipped in beaten egg, then crumbs).

To pan-fry:

1. Brown meat on both sides in a small amount of fat in a heavy skillet.
2. Season with salt and pepper and turn occasionally. Do not cover, do not add liquid. Serve as soon as tender.

To deep-fat fry (French fry):

1. Use your electric fryer or heavy sauce pot with enough fat to completely cover the meat or croquettes. Pieces of meat should be of even size. Coat meat with egg and crumbs or batter.
2. Heat shortening to 375°.
3. Fry a few pieces at a time, without crowding fryer, just long enough to brown and cook through.
4. Drain on soft paper and keep hot until served.

How to Stew Meats

1. Cut the meat into uniform pieces (about 1 1/2 inches across). For brown stew, flour them and season with salt and pepper. For light stew just season, omitting flour.
2. Brown the meat well in a small amount of fat (omit this step for a light stew).
3. Barely cover the meat with water, put a cover on the pot and cook at a simmer until meat is tender, 2 1/2 to 3 hours. Vegetables (any kind that suits your fancy) may be added the last 30 to 35 minutes.
4. Thicken stew if it isn't thickened from the flour used for browning. Mix flour or cornstarch to a paste in cold water for thickening, using 1 tablespoon cornstarch or 2 of flour for 1 cup liquid in the pot.
5. Many variations in seasonings are possible. Tomato juice or wine is often used for part of the liquid. Herbs and spices may be added to the simmering stew.

How to Simmer Meats

Many large pieces not naturally tender are cooked this way. Just cover the meat with water and cook under the boiling point as long as necessary to tenderize.

How To Thaw Frozen Meats

At room temperature, if you are in a hurry. In the refrigerator if there's time. Don't do it in water unless you are cooking it in the same water; you'll lose too much good meat flavor. Either completely unwrap or loosen wrappings on meat thawing.

POULTRY

How to Store Poultry

Keep frozen poultry frozen until you are ready to use it. Once thawed, cook it immediately. Don't ever refreeze it. (After cooking, you may freeze part of the cooked meat, if you wish.)

Don't keep a fresh bird more than a day or two before cooking. Cover the fresh poultry loosely and store it in the coldest part of the refrigerator (not the freezer, necessarily).

Cooked poultry meat should be refrigerated as soon as possible—don't let it sit around at room temperature after dinner. It should be eaten within 3 or 4 days. Poultry that has been around too long, cooked or uncooked, can cause serious food poisoning.

Never roast a chicken, turkey, or other bird halfway one day, finishing it the next. **Never** stuff a bird a day or two early or stuff it before freezing. **Such practices encourage the development of harmful bacteria in poultry and stuffings.**

How to Broil Chicken

A broiler weighing from 1 to 1 1/2 pounds will take about half an hour's cooking. This size should be split to make two servings. A larger broiler, preferably not over 2 pounds, can be quartered to serve four.

Brush the chicken all over with soft butter or other fat and lay on a rack about 6 inches from the broiling unit with heat at moderate temperature. Broil 20 minutes on the cut side, then season with salt and pepper, turn and broil 10 minutes longer, or until nicely browned and tender. Season and serve on a hot platter with the drippings or with a sauce or gravy made using the giblets.

Small split broilers can be broiled until brown on the skin side, then filled with moist dressing made with crumbs, chopped giblets, seasonings, and a little butter and water or stock and finished in a 325° oven, with or without a cover on the pan.

How to Fry Chicken
Chicken may be fried in deep or shallow fat, with or without a coating. The usual method is this: Shake the pieces of chicken in a paper bag with flour and seasonings, then brown them without crowding the pan in 1/2 inch hot shortening. Don't use butter or margarine, as it scorches too easily. Turn the chicken frequently and reduce heat after browning. Cook uncovered about 45 minutes or until the chicken is very tender. If the fryer is over 3 1/2 pounds, cover the skillet after reducing the heat following browning and let the meat steam tender. Chicken may be finished in a moderate 325° oven.

Oven-fried chicken: This is very easy. Heat 1/2 inch fat (butter or bacon fat) in your roasting pan, lay chicken pieces (floured and seasoned) in a single layer without crowding. Bake at 375° for 45 minutes to 1 hour, turning just once.

How to Roast Chicken
Wipe chicken inside and out with a damp cloth, remove any pinfeathers, and season inside with salt and pepper. Cut out oil sac on back of tail. Stuff the chicken with any favorite dressing, filling the neck as well as the body cavity. Skewer neck skin to back to hold the stuffing and lace the larger opening with cord over small steel skewers. Tie drumsticks to tail with cord. Brush all over with soft butter and place on a rack in an open roasting pan. Roast at 325°. Breast and drumsticks may be covered with aluminum foil or fat-saturated cheesecloth to keep them from drying out. Use no water in the roasting pan.

How to Stew Chicken
Stew chicken whole or in pieces. Cover with water, add-

ing 1 1/2 teaspoons salt, an onion, a small carrot, a rib of celery, and a few whole peppercorns. Cover and simmer until meat is tender, 2 to 4 hours, depending on age and size of chicken. Chill the broth; remove fat for cooking purposes and strain the broth. You have a cooked chicken for a stew with dumplings or for one of a hundred chicken dishes plus stock for soup, sauce, or gravy.

KINDS AND TYPES OF TURKEY AVAILABLE

The broiler-fryer. From 4 to 8 pounds, this is for a small group. These plump birds look like broad-breasted chickens and may be stuffed and roasted, broiled, baked, fried, or prepared in any way you would fix chicken. They come ready to cook and are beautiful little birds, very flavorsome.

Roasting turkey. There's no substitute for your old favorite, the big bird on Thanksgiving and Christmas. From 8 to 24 pounds, there's a size for everyone.

Half turkey, quarter turkey. A half bird can be roasted with dressing. It can make a very handsome appearance on the serving platter. Usually it weighs from 4 to 15 pounds. A half turkey weighing 15 pounds will have a huge, meaty breast that will yield dozens of wide slices of white meat. A quarter turkey weighs around 3 1/2 to 7 pounds and includes either drumstick or wing. It is roasted, as a rule.

Frozen stuffed turkey. This 8 to 12 pounder is stuffed with old-fashioned herb or corn-bread filling. Always cook from frozen state and follow packer's directions.

Turkey breast rack and rolled breast of turkey. These are choice roasts. The breast rack has the bone in. Poultry-cooking experts believe that the bone contributes to the flavor of the roast turkey meat as does the skin. The boned roll is compact; the skin is drawn up and sewed around it. This form is available in some markets.

Turkey roll. The cooked, boned frozen meat of turkey shaped into a roll for slicing is used extensively by institutions for sandwiches and casserole dishes.

Cut-up turkey. This is sold by the piece, like chicken.

You may buy wings, thighs, drumsticks, breasts, giblets, and so forth. Wings may be divided into wing tips, flat wings, and wing sticks. Don't underestimate turkey wings as a good dinner. They're meaty and fine flavored.

Smoked turkey. This is the epicure's dish. It is expensive, rich-bodied meat, highly valued as cocktail food, especially. Comes whole or half, cooked and ready to eat.

Canned turkey. You can buy boneless turkey in 6- or 7-ounce cans and in bigger ones weighing 1 to 2 1/4 pounds. Any recipe calling for cooked turkey can use this kind of meat. Canned turkey with noodles, smoked turkey, and smoked turkey pâté are a few of the specialty items in cans.

How to Store Turkey and How Long to Keep It
Fresh turkey will wait two or three days for roasting, if you keep it loosely wrapped in the refrigerator. If you should buy your bird with head and feet on, undrawn, be sure to draw the turkey and clean the giblets right away. No bird should be stored with its insides in.

Frozen turkey, except the stuffed one, should be defrosted. It will take from 2 to 3 days to defrost the average turkey in the refrigerator in its original wrappings. You can defrost the bird under cold running water in 4 to 6 hours. Cook it promptly after defrosting. Do not refreeze once thawed (but you can freeze it again after roasting).

Cooked turkey should be used within 4 days if not frozen. If you freeze the meat, it will keep several months. Never leave roasted turkey out of the refrigerator after the meal. As soon as you've finished, strip the meat from the bones and freeze it or store it in covered containers. Breast meat and thigh meat may be stored separately. Scraps can be packed by themselves for use in casseroles.

Crack the bones and boil them for soup to use soon or for concentrated stock to be frozen. Remove stuffing to refrigerator dishes or freezer. Frozen stuffing may be kept a month. Use it within a day or two if not frozen. Turkey gravy should be refrigerated promptly.

How to Cook Turkey by the Piece
Roast a turkey breast or half breast or a boned turkey

breast; braise other parts, that is, brown them, then add a little liquid, cover, and cook until tender.

A turkey of 24 to 30 pounds cuts to yield four to six servings for a half breast, four servings to a whole leg, about two servings per drumstick or thigh. A wing serves one nicely, 1 or 2 wingsticks make a serving portion. Thaw frozen parts before cooking.

How to Roast a Half Breast of Turkey
Rub the cavity with salt. Draw up the neck skin with a large needle and cord, making a pocket. Lace across the cavity, catching skin at each side. Insert heavy paper under the lacing to form a side wall for the stuffing.

Hold the breast piece neck down and stuff it loosely with 2 to 3 cups of stuffing. Stuffing absorbs moisture from the turkey and swells as it cooks. Finish lacing over the paper, drawing up the skin to protect the meat.

If the wing has been left on, sew it tight to the body or fasten it down with small poultry pins stuck in at an angle. If the piece has no wing, sew or skewer the flap of skin and meat to the breast meat. Grease the skin. Roast the half breast paperside down on a rack in an open pan at 325° for 3 1/2 to 4 1/2 hours, depending on size. Baste with butter several times. Or protect with butter-saturated cheesecloth or aluminum foil, as you do a whole turkey.

FATS

Bacon, Ham, and Chicken Fat
These three fats are excellent shortenings, and they do lend a flavor of their own, as a rule. Use bacon or ham drippings to season any green vegetable and to fry chicken (with some shortening, too, because of the salt content and low-smoking point). Any of these three fats is good in muffins, corn bread, waffles, pancakes. Chicken fat makes an excellent base for a cream sauce or stock sauce to use on cooked chicken, veal, or in vegetable dishes.

Cooking Fats and Frying
There are two kinds of frying: in shallow fat, called pan frying or sautéing; in deep fat, called deep-fat frying or French frying. The all-purpose shortenings and oils are equal-

ly suitable. Butter and margarine are suitable for pan frying or sautéing foods that cook quickly. These fats break down and scorch readily, so many cooks don't consider them suitable for longer frying jobs.

Both shortenings and oils, except olive oil, are suited to deep-fat frying, too. A high smoking point is a requirement for deep-fat frying. Any fat that breaks down at a temperature of 350° is unsuitable. That eliminates butter, margarine, drippings, and chicken fat.

How to Care for Frying Fat

Don't leave it in your fryer. Cool it to a safe handling temperature and strain it through several layers of cheesecloth to remove all the foreign particles, such as bits of batter or coating from fried food. Remove sediment from the cooker and wash it well. Return strained fat to its can and add a little fresh shortening while it is still warm. This freshens and prolongs the life of the frying fat. Store fat in a cool, dark place until you need it again.

To clarify frying fat that is beginning to break down (getting dark, with off-odor or flavor), slice raw potatoes into it and heat gradually. The potato will remove odor and flavor. Discard the spuds. Don't even try to clarify fat that is really dark and rancid smelling. It has deteriorated to a point beyond help.

Rules for French Frying

1. Use electric fryer or heavy saucepan with straight sides and some kind of frying basket, plus deep-fat thermometer.
2. Fill cooker not more than one-third to one-half full of shortening or oil.
3. Set frying basket in cooker and attach thermometer if you are using a saucepan. Heat fat to proper temperature for your food.
4. Immerse food (don't crowd basket) and cook for proper time.
5. Lift out and drain on absorbent paper.
6. Serve hot.

FISH

How to Cook Fish

In the oven.   Any kind of fish, any size, stuffed or un-stuffed, in steaks or fillets, may be baked. The general rule is this: Use a 400° oven and bake only until the fish flakes. The time averages around 11 to 15 minutes per pound.

Whole fish should be cleaned and scaled for baking, but the head may be left on. Wash in cold salt water and dry with paper towels. If you stuff the fish, sprinkle with salt and pepper. Fill loosely and sew or skewer the opening. (Insert metal skewers or toothpicks every inch, across the opening, and lace with string or coarse thread.) To facilitate removal from the pan to the serving platter, place the fish on oiled brown paper, waxed paper, buttered cheesecloth, or foil for baking. Or bake on a heatproof platter. Brush with butter or lay bacon strips over the fish. You may try these:

1. Rolling the fish in grated cheese or coating with mayon-naise and cheese before baking.

2. Basting it with white wine or sour cream as it bakes.

3. Marinating it in French dressing for 1 or 2 hours before baking.

Fillets and steaks are brushed with butter or coated with crumbs and placed in a shallow baking dish. Sometimes they're baked in a sauce, in which case the oven temperature usually is 375° and baking takes about 25 minutes.

Hot oven method for fillets.   Many cooks favor the al-most instantaneous hot oven method of cooking egged and crumbed fillets of any kind. The oven is preheated to 550°, the well-coated fillets are laid out in a shallow baking pan and popped into the oven for just about 8 minutes. They cook and brown nicely in that time, and there's no fish odor in the kitchen.

In the broiler.   This is a favorite method for steaks and fillets, for whole small fish without stuffing, and for split fish under 4 pounds. It couldn't be easier or quicker. Use high heat (550°) and broil 2 to 3 inches from heat. Brush with butter or mayonnaise or dredge in egg and fine crumbs, then brush with butter. Turn steaks, split and whole fish (except sole and flounder) once with a spatula during broiling. . Fillets are thinner, so broil them skin-side down and don't try to turn them. Season after broiling with salt and pepper and serve with lemon or a sauce. Thick steaks and whole fish are basted with butter several times during broiling, especially cod, striped bass, and halibut. One basting is a good idea for fillets, although not really necessary.

At this high heat and close proximity to the broiling unit, fish cooks fast, becomes golden brown, retains all its flavor, and has no fishy odor. Fillets take 5 to 10 minutes, depending on thickness; steaks 6 to 12 minutes. If you start them frozen, they take a few minutes longer. Watch the broiling carefully. Overcooked fish becomes tough and dry.

In the pan. Small dressed fish, steaks, and fillets may be pan fried. Use shortening, bacon fat, oil, or a combination of butter or margarine and one of these fats. Have the skillet (a roomy one) very hot and the fat 1/8 inch deep. Coat the fish with flour or with beaten egg and crumbs or cornmeal and brown quickly on each side, turning once. Season with salt and pepper on turning or after cooking. Fish flakes when done. Don't overcook. Serve with lemon quarters and tartar sauce.

In deep fat. Small fish such as smelts, moderately small ones such as lake perch, fish fillets of many kinds, croquettes, and fish balls are cooked this way. Dip in milk or beaten egg, then in fine crumbs or cornmeal. Use a frying basket. Don't crowd the fish. Fry in a kettle half-full of shortening at a temperature of 375°, using a deep-fat thermometer if you haven't an electric French fryer with controlled heat. Three to 5 minutes should be enough, just long enough for beautiful browning. Drain on paper towels and sprinkle with salt and pepper. Serve with lemon quarters and tartar sauce.

SHELLFISH

Clams and Clambakes
Clams are at the height of their popularity during the summer months when their cousins the oysters aren't much in evidence. But they're available the year round for eating

on the half shell, in chowders, and, in New England especially, for eating as steamed clams.

On the West Coast as well as the East, thousands of clam diggers gather their own shellfish. There are many more varieties of clams to be had than ever reach the commercial markets.

Along the Eastern Coast clams coming to market are the hard-shell, soft-shell, and surf. Western varieties include soft-shell, butter, razor, and pismo clams—the last a one-and-a-half pounder. Littleneck and cherrystone clams from the East Coast are merely the small sizes, the on-the-half-shell clams of the hard-clam variety. Their older brothers and sisters are known as chowder clams. "Steamers" are the little ones of the soft-shells, the meltingly tender clambake clams, so prized by New Englanders.

Before You Start to Cook Clams

Make sure you get fresh ones. Fresh hard-shell clams, like fresh oysters, have tightly closed shells. If the shell gapes, discard the clam. With other varieties some constriction of the neck or siphon when touched is an indication that the clam is alive.

To get sand out of clams, put them in fresh water for about 3 hours before using and sprinkle a handful of cornmeal over them. The clams will absorb the meal and expel the sand they're harboring. Or cover the clams with clean sea water or brine made with 1/3 cup salt to 1 gallon tap water and let stand 15 to 20 minutes. The clams will open and discharge sand. Change the water and do this again several times. Then wash and steam your clams.

How to Cook Clams

In steam. Use soft-shell or "steamer" clams, 15 to 25 per portion. Wash under running water. Place in a large kettle with very little water. Cover and steam 8 to 12 minutes or until the shells partially open. Serve at once with individual dishes of melted butter. Or use the clams for a prepared dish. Some people also like a little lemon juice either in the butter or provided as a wedge of lemon.

The liquor left in the kettle is clam broth, as much relished as the clams themselves. It may be strained and sipped, or the clams may be dipped in it, then into butter. Steamed clams are eaten with the fingers, not forks, and if bibs aren't provided, large napkins should be.

In the oven.   A half pound of clams in the shell per person, at least. Wash well and roast in a shallow baking pan at 450° until the shells open, about 15 minutes. Serve them immediately with lots of butter.

How-To's with Boiled Lobster

How to choose and cook it.   A 1-pound chicken lobster makes a good individual serving. If you have a crowd, buy them bigger. If the lobster meat is to be removed from the shell and prepared with a sauce, a 2-pound lobster should make 2 or 3 servings.

Get a kettle big enough to hold all your lobsters with room to spare or do the cooking in installments or in two containers. Fill the container almost half full of water and add 1 tablespoon salt per quart. When the salt water is boiling, grasp the lobster behind the head and drop it headfirst into the water. Cover and heat to quick boil, then simmer 20 minutes. Drain and serve at once with lots of melted butter, or cool and remove the meat to use as you wish.

All the lobster meat is edible except the eye and small sac behind it attached to the intestinal vein. The green liver, or tomalley, which fills most of the body cavity, is particularly delicious. It may be mixed with melted butter and used as a dunk for the lobster meat or added to a sauce if the lobster is to be served in sauce.

How to serve it.   Provide a nutcracker for cracking the claws and a small seafood fork for each person and supply melted butter in a little dish for dunking. Potato chips and pickles are all that lobster lovers require in addition. But give them bibs or big napkins.

How to eat it.

1. Twist off the claws and crack them with a nutcracker, pliers, or even a rock. Pick out the meat and eat it.

2. Separate the tailpiece from the body by arching the back until it cracks.

3. Bend back the tailpiece and break off the flippers. Insert a fork at the point where you broke the flippers and push out the meat. Dunk it in butter and eat it.

4. Unhinge the back from the body, after eating the green liver. Open the remaining part of the body by cracking it apart sideways. There is some good meat in this section, but you have to work for it.

5. Suck the meat from the small claws.

How to Broil a Live Lobster

Place the lobster on its back on your cutting board, being sure his large claws are plugged. Cross these and hold firmly with the left hand. Draw a deep breath and insert the point of a sharp, heavy knife between the body shell and tail segment; cut down to break spinal cord. Split from head to tail; open lobster flat. Remove the sac behind the eyes and the intestinal vein. Everything else is edible. Crack the claws with a mallet. Brush all exposed flesh with melted butter, place on a greased rack and broil flesh-side up 8 to 10 minutes; turn, cook 6 to 8 minutes longer. Provide melted butter and big napkins.

If you aren't serving the liver with the lobster, use it in some other seafood dish and fill the cavity with fine buttered crumbs mixed with a little grated onion and a dash of Worcestershire sauce. Or mix the liver with butter crumbs, salt, pepper, and a dash of Worcestershire, and return to the shell for broiling.

What To Do with Lobster Tails

Boil them. If you have time, thaw the tails before cooking. Place them in a kettle of rapidly boiling salted water (1 teaspoon salt per quart) and bring again to the boiling point. Then lower the heat to a simmer and simmer 1 minute per ounce, plus 1 minute "for the pot." Thus you'd cook an 8-ounce tail 9 minutes, a 12-ounce tail 13 minutes, and a baby 4-ounce tail 5 minutes.

If you start them frozen, you'll have to add 2 minutes to your cooking time. To keep them straight (they curl in cooking) insert skewers lengthwise before you put the tails into the pot.

Eat these boiled lobster tails hot with melted butter, cold with mayonnaise, or remove the meat from the shell, cut it into chunks, and turn it into salad, casserole, or another lobster treat.

How to get the meat out of the shell: Take a pair of kitchen scissors and cut right down the middle of the underpart, get your fingers in there and pull out the cooked meat in one piece.

Broil them. Split the tail in half lengthwise, after thawing. Brush well with melted butter or margarine and place flesh-side up on broiler rack about 4 inches from the heat. Broil 8 to 10 minutes or until tinged with brown. The shell turns coral during cooking, as with boiled lobster. Serve at once with lots of butter and a slice of lemon.

Precook frozen tails in salted water 5 minutes before broiling. If you prefer not to split the tails, either trim away the undershell with scissors and loosen the flesh slightly from the sides or split down the back with a sharp knife or scissors and open out the tail. If you cut away the membrane, grasp the tail in both hands and bend it backward toward the shell-side to crack and prevent curling during cooking.

Or bake them in foil. Thaw the tails and cut away the undershells. Brush with butter, wrap well in foil, and bake on a baking sheet at 450° for 25 minutes for tails up to and including 8 ounces, 30 minutes for tails to 12 ounces, and 35 minutes for tails up to 1 pound in weight.

How to Cook Shrimp
Buy a pound to serve three or four people; in general, 1 1/2 pounds yield 3/4 pound ready-to-eat meat, after shelling, cooking, and deveining.

Drop the shrimps into salted boiling water (1 quart water and 1/4 cup salt for 1 1/2 pounds shrimp). Cover, return to boiling point, and simmer 5 minutes. Drain, peel, remove sand veins, and chill to use as you wish. Too cook peeled shrimps, follow the same method, but reduce the amount of salt (2 tablespoons for 1 1/2 pounds).

EGGS

How to Use Frozen Eggs

If you haven't a way to use a dozen egg yolks after making angel cake, freeze them. Egg whites freeze even more easily, and whole eggs may be frozen out of the shell.

To freeze whites. Merely freeze at 0° or below in packages of a useful size, for example, enough whites for an angel cake or for a meringue pie topping. Don't mix them. They'll whip beautifully when thawed.

. To freeze egg yolks. To prevent a rubbery texture, you'll have to add sugar, corn syrup, or salt, depending on how you are going to use the yolks. Sweet ones are fine for cakes, custards, puddings; salty ones for scrambled eggs. Stir yolks just enough to break them, but don't incorporate air. Add 1 teaspoon salt or 2 teaspoons sugar, or 1 tablespoon syrup to 1 pint yolks.

To freeze whole eggs. Stir them lightly, as for yolks alone, adding salt or sweetening. Or freeze whole, individually, by breaking into muffin cups lined with paper baking cups or into ice-cube trays with dividers. Freeze solid, then package enough for one use in a plastic bag.

How to Fry Eggs

Heat bacon, ham, or sausage drippings, butter or margarine to coat the bottom of a skillet big enough to hold the eggs without crowding. Break eggs one by one into a saucer and slip them from the saucer into the hot fat. (This procedure prevents you from spoiling the skilletful of eggs with a rare, but possible poor egg and also keeps out of the pan the yolk you've just put your thumb into). When egg whites have begun to set, pour 1/2 eggshell of water into the skillet with the eggs and cover them. Turn off the heat and let the eggs stand a few seconds until the yolks have filmed over. Season with salt and pepper and lift with a broad spatula to hot plates.

Or, leave all the fat from the bacon or sausage in the skillet, get it hot and slip the eggs, singly, into it. They curl and puff a bit, but look attractive. Then spoon hot fat over the yolks until they are as set as you like them. These are sometimes known as "basted" eggs.

How to Hard-Cook or Soft-Cook Eggs

The hard-boiled egg shouldn't be boiled, only simmered. Boiling makes it tough. Place the eggs in a deep saucepan and add enough cold water to cover them. Set over moderate heat and bring rapidly to boiling. Then turn off heat and cover for 2 minutes for very soft eggs; 4 minutes for medium soft eggs; 15 minutes for hard-cooked eggs. Remove the eggs from the water with a tablespoon. If you are cooking more than 4 eggs at once, don't turn off the heat, but keep water below simmering for 4 to 6 minutes for soft or medium eggs, 20 minutes for hard-cooked eggs.

Cool hard-cooked eggs under cold water to prevent formation of a green sulphur ring around the yolks, if you are using the eggs in a prepared dish instead of eating them hot. This also makes them easier to shell.

How to Broil Eggs

Slip the broken eggs into a hot skillet with a little melted butter in it. Place over low heat until eggs begin to set. Pour melted butter over the tops and place under the broiler, turned low. Cook until the yolks are as firm as wanted, 2 to 4 minutes. The butter will brown somewhat under the broiler and the eggs will have a rich, buttery flavor. Grated cheese or 1 tablespoon cream per egg may be added before the eggs go under the broiler.

How to Scramble Eggs

There are almost as many opinions about the proper way to scramble eggs as there are about the best way to make coffee. One cook likes to serve soft, creamy, moist eggs, so she does the scrambling over hot water. Another likes to see brown color on scrambled eggs and insists that the only way to do this job is in a well-buttered skillet over direct heat.

Add milk, add water, add wine, add nothing at all, just scramble them. Put in cheese, put in chives, drop in some onion or ham or flaked fish. Scramble in butter, scramble in bacon fat.

Too much heat or prolonged cooking by any method is ruinous to the delicate texture of eggs.

How to Poach Eggs

Poached eggs are the foundation of many famous dishes,

but for breakfast they are best plain. Bring about 2 inches of water in a shallow pan to boiling. Turn down the heat to hold at simmering. Break an egg at a time into a saucer and slip quickly into the water. Cook 3 to 5 minutes, depending on the firmness you like. Remove eggs with a slotted spoon and serve on toast or in one of many ways. Eggs may be poached in tomato juice, cream, milk, dry white wine, or chicken broth. Salt and vinegar are not necessary.

HOW TO COOK MACARONI, SPAGHETTI, AND NOODLES

Bring 3 quarts of water to boil in a large kettle, add 1 tablespoon salt, and the macaroni product. Boil uncovered until tender, 8 to 10 minutes or longer (follow package directions). Drain. If you cook more than 8 ounces of the macaroni at a time, you'll need more water and salt.

Macaroni products double in bulk during cooking. Cook 1 pound of macaroni for 6 to 8 servings, 8 ounces for 3 to 6 servings. How much you need depends upon what you combine with the product.

RICE

Kinds of Rice Available

White milled rice. This is the common rice, and it comes long grain, medium grain, and short grain. The long grain is more expensive than the others since it breaks rather easily and thus requires more care in handling. All these grains are rice with the outer bran coat removed.

Brown rice. A little darker than white rice, it is the same thing but includes the bran coat and germ of the grain, which makes it more nutritious. It takes somewhat longer to cook and keeps less well than the snowy rice.

Precooked rice. This is long-grain rice prepared so that it may be brought to a boil, removed from the heat, and be ready for the table. Naturally, you pay a little more for it, but it is a great convenience to a cook who is in a hurry.

Converted rice. A special process forces the water-soluble B vitamins into the center of the grain. It is more nutritious than white rice and not nearly so white. It costs a little more, too.

Wild rice. Not really rice at all, but the seed of a marsh grass. The grains are long, dark, and greenish, chewier when cooked than other rice. Wild rice has to be gathered by hand, and thus it is always expensive. It is considered a delicacy when served as an accompaniment or stuffing of game.

How to Cook Rice

To get fluffy, white, and tender rice in no time, simply follow these directions. Put 1 cup rice, 2 cups cold water, and 1 teaspoon salt into a 2-quart saucepan with a tight-fitting lid. Set over high heat until the rice boils vigorously. Reduce heat as low as possible and let rice steam about 14 minutes longer or until all the water is absorbed and the grains are fluffy and separate. Remove the cover and let the rice steam dry and fluffy. Do not stir rice as it cooks. If necessary, lift with a fork to keep it from sticking. Rice triples in bulk when cooked. Remember that when planning servings.

WHAT TO DO WITH UNUSED FOODS

Meats, Poultry, Fish

Bake in a casserole with noodles, spaghetti, or rice and a can of cream of mushroom, cream of chicken, or cream of celery soup. Cut into julienne strips for a chef's salad; dice for a meat, fish, or poultry salad, which could take a leftover hard-cooked egg or two, along with its celery, pickle, and dressing. Grind and mix with potatoes for hash. Mince, season with onion and salad dressing for sandwiches. Cream and serve on hot biscuits or baked potatoes. Chop, add onion, celery, and gravy, thick white sauce or undiluted cream soup; spread on rolled biscuit dough, roll up, bake, then slice and serve hot with cream sauce or more gravy.

Eggs

Leftover egg whites can always be used for white cake, angel cake, a meringue topping for pie. But what of spare yolks? Drop them carefully into hot water, cook firm, then chill to use in salads or vegetable casseroles. Or cream with dried beef and serve on toast. Grate to garnish soup or salad. Mash, mix with salad dressing for sandwich filling. A few yolks may be scrambled with more whole eggs, but scrambled yolks alone aren't very tender. Whole hard-cooked eggs make excellent casseroles and can be creamed with vegetables, meat, poultry, or fish. Leftover poached, fried, and scrambled eggs can be smoothed in your electric blender for soup along with vegetables and perhaps cooked bacon.

Rice

A little leftover rice makes a wonderful salad with diced chicken (canned, maybe?) chutney, mayonnaise. Or turn it into "heavenly hash" with bits of fruit, diced marshmallow, whipped cream. Or add to meat loaf mixture, meat soup.

Vegetables

Add sharp French dressing or mayonnaise to leftover vegetables before refrigerating them for use in a salad. They may be mixed with greens, other cooked vegetables, or vegetables and meats. Puree in a blender and use in cream soup. Cream with other vegetables, or tuck into casserole dishes. Baked beans may be blended into soup.

Mashed potatoes make potato cakes. Just shape into patties, brown in butter. Or whip mashed spuds light with milk and an egg and brown atop a meat stew; or drop in puffs onto a greased cooky sheet and brown in the oven. Or add enough flour to make mashed potatoes rollable, roll into a rectangle, cover with creamed meat, fish, or poultry, roll like jelly roll, brush with butter, and bake. Mashed potatoes make wonderful cream of potato soup and can even make potato salad, with dressing, celery, pickles, and onion. Mashed sweet potatoes can be whipped smooth, mounded on pineapple rings, brushed with butter and baked to serve with chops.

Fruits

Fruit leftovers seldom are much of a problem. Combine them with other fruits for salad, fruit cup, jellied salads, and desserts. Use with crumbs in bread- or cake-crumb puddings. Chop and serve as a pudding or ice-cream sauce. Fruit juices and syrups, especially from canned fruits, can be used for pudding sauces or sauce for baked or broiled ham. Muffins, pancakes, and waffles can have fruit in them or in sauces for them.

Breads

Toast makes croutons for soup. Crushed crumbs can go into casserole toppings, stuffings, bread puddings. Stale doughnuts and raisin bread may be used for a kind of fruit betty. Crumble them, moisten with milk and a beaten egg or two, add brown sugar, a little cinnamon, whatever canned or dried fruits you have on hand, bake brown, and eat with cream—good!

Cakes and Cookies

Sprinkle coarse pieces or split layers of stale cake with sherry, put together with soft custard or cream filling to make a delightful pudding or revived cream-filled cake. Cut strips of angel food, chiffon, or sponge cake, roll in sweetened condensed milk or honey, then in coconut or chopped nuts, bake or broil and serve as tea cakes. Combine cooky or cake crumbs with crushed pineapple, whipped cream, and marshmallow pieces and serve in sherbet cups. Oven-dry stale cake, crumble fine, and use with raisins or nuts and butter as a coffe-cake filling or topping.

FROZEN FOODS

Frozen foods have many factors worth considering. They are convenient, economical, and are easy to use timesavers. The amount needed to prepare a meal can be easily determined by the size of package or portion control package, available at your local market. Fruits, vegetables, and fish are available regardless of the season.

Many items are packed by different companies in the country. You may find that certain items packed by a particular company appeal to your taste or need. It is safe to assume that the item you are purchasing is of the highest quality.

Once you've made the purchase, care must be taken to keep these foods under proper freezing temperatures. Low temperature is necessary. Frozen foods must be stored at 0° F or lower. Too long storage of food may cause loss of quality.

Foods that have been partially thawed can be safely refrozen if they still feel cold, if ice crystals are still on them, or if they have been thawed for only a short time. If food has been thawed for a long period of time and you are doubtful about safety of it, do not serve.

Refreezing raw fish when thawed is not recommended. Fish when thawed completely before cooking loses much of its water content. Do not thaw frozen fish completely. When rolling, flour, eggs, and crumbs will adhere to fish if only partially thawed.

Recommended Storage Periods for Meat at 0° F

Storage period in months	Kind of meat
9–12 months	Beef, lamb, and veal, not ground
4–6 months	Fresh pork, not ground; all ground meats except pork
3–4 months	All variety meats, except pork livers
2–3 months	Smoked ham or pork; bacon slab; unsalted, ground pork; smoked and seasoned sausage; wieners with skins
1–2 months	Pork livers; pork links; sausage seasoned and salted, not smoked; sliced bacon (not recommended)

Vegetables

Vegetables such as peas or beans to be frozen should be picked when at their peak ripeness. To ensure peak flavor handle as quickly as possible. Use an aluminum, enamel, or stainless steel kettle to blanch.

Vegetables are high in vitamins and minerals when picked from the garden. To ensure the nutritional value in vegetables, care must be taken to preserve them from the time they are picked until they are served.

Cook vegetables in a small amount of water. Frozen vegetables require less cooking time than fresh, due to the blanching in the freezing process. Do not overcook. Frozen vegetables and fruits retain their natural color. Hold cooked frozen vegetables in steam pan or kettle for as short a time as possible. Long standing tends to lower the quality and texture and also loses color and flavor.

Shell peas, Green beans. Blanch in boiling water, if small 45 to 50 seconds, large 60 seconds, or until water comes to a boil. Use a wire rack for blanching. If you don't have a wire rack, drain in a colander, immersing the colander and peas in ice-cube water for 3 to 4 minutes. Drain well. Pack in plastic containers or heavy plastic bags. Allow 1/2 inch of space on top of the container.

Beans: Green, Wax, or Snap Beans. Wash beans, cut into desired lengths or slices. Blanch in boiling water. Chill in cold water 3 to 5 minutes. Drain well. Pack in containers, leaving space on top.

Beets. Wash beets well. Cook until tender. Cool, peel, and pack into desired size containers. If small, young beets, freeze whole. Cube, slice, or use serrated knife to cut large beets.

Green peppers, red hot peppers. May be blanched. If used in salads, freeze without blanching. These can also be used in casserole dishes.

Asparagus. Trim bottom spears, cut into desired length. Blanch about 4 minutes. Chill in ice water 4 minutes. Drain. Lay on cookie sheet, freeze, pack quickly in plastic containers or heavy plastic bags.

Pumpkin. Cut up pumpkin, remove shell and seeds. Cook until well done. Mash. Cool and pack in freezer cartons, allowing 1/2 inch space on top of carton.

Fruits

Sugar Pack. Place berries in a shallow container, add 3/4 cup sugar per quart of berries. Freeze.

Syrup Pack. Mix 4 cups cold water and 2 cups sugar until sugar is dissolved. Freeze.

Blackberries, boysenberries, loganberries, raspberries. Use sugar pack.

Blueberries, elderberries, huckleberries. Use fully ripened berries. These berries may be packed in syrup or mixed with 1/2 to 3/4 cup sugar. Mix gently to draw juice. Pack berries in freezer containers. Allow space, about 1/2 inch from top.

Strawberries. Berries should be firm, not overripe.

Wash berries before hulling. Strawberries may be packed whole, cut in halves, or crushed to be used on ice cream desserts. Whole berries may be frozen in syrup.

Cantaloupe. Melons should be firm and well ripened. Cut in cubes or balls. Cover with syrup pack. Allow space. Freeze the same as other fruits.

Baked Goods

All baked goods can be frozen satisfactorily. The only exception is popovers. These are best served shortly after baking. Make certain that all baked goods are completely cooled before freezing; otherwise you may have a soggy product. To simplify reheating, wrap in wrapper or container that can be put directly in the oven.

Partially baked homemade rolls and bread can be kept in your freezer from 6 to 8 months. They need not be thawed completely before popping in the oven to finish baking and are delicious when served hot.

Pies may be frozen baked or unbaked. To keep the edge of the pie crust from breaking, freeze the pie first. Remove it from the freezer, cover with a paper pie plate, and wrap securely in foil wrap or moisture-proof wrap. Return to the freezer as quickly as possible. Reheat in the oven when ready to serve. Unbaked pies may be put directly in the oven from the freezer.

Freeze cookies on a flat pan before packaging. This will prevent breakage and sticking together when packaged in bags. Return to freezer as quickly as possible. If polyethylene bags are used for packaging cookies, for safety use double bags. This prevents the cookies from drying out or acquiring freezer taste.

Fruit cakes baked ahead as gifts may be kept in the freezer for months. Fruit cakes grow more mellow with longer storage.

After removing products from the freezer, allow them to thaw out completely at room temperature before unwrapping.

To successfully freeze bread or roll dough, double the

amount of yeast. This should be a rich dough; freeze immediately after kneading and mixing. Store dough in cartons and containers, the amount you wish to use. When ready to use, allow 2 or 3 hours to thaw. Remove dough from container, place in greased mixing bowl. When raised, shape into rolls, buns, or coffee cakes. The dough will keep in the freezer several months.

Freeze your own bake-and-serve rolls. Bake rolls at 300°F about 20 to 30 minutes. Rolls should still be pale. Cool before freezing. To avoid crushing, do not pack too tightly. Thaw in container unopened 10 to 15 minutes, or until thawed. Bake in a hot oven (400°F) for 5 to 10 minutes.

Frozen Pizza. When making pizza and the recipe is too large for your immediate use, make up a whole pizza, then freeze one half. Bake one half ready to serve. Bake the other half just long enough to set crust, without the sausage, mushrooms, or olives. Add these when ready to serve.

Cake. Bake the cake, but frost only as much as you need. Cut the rest in smaller portions, cool well. Wrap in foil wrap or store in cans or plastic containers. Mark and freeze. Thaw before frosting.

Soups and Casseroles

When recipes are for quantity cooking, freeze soups for future use in freezer cartons in the amounts you will need.

If you can spare individual casserole dishes or large ones, freeze extra casseroles. You'll be glad you did for that emergency or very busy day.

SOME VARIATIONS OF TOAST FOR MEALS

For all these, trim crusts or leave them. Cut toast in halves or in triangular quarters.

Brown-sugar toast. Cream together 1/4 cup butter and 1/2 cup brown sugar. Add 1 tablespoon cream, and, if you like, a little cinnamon or grated lemon rind. Spread on toasted bread, place on a cooky sheet, and broil until bubbly. Enough for 6 slices of toast.

Cheese toast. Butter toast and sprinkle with grated cheese—Cheddar, Swiss, Italian type, or whatever you like— and bake 3 minutes or broil until cheese melts. Good with a salad luncheon.

Cinnamon toast. Butter toast as thickly as you like and sprinkle with cinnamon and sugar (1 teaspoon cinnamon to 1/4 cup sugar). Broil 1 minute or place in 350° oven for 3 minutes.

Fried toast. All you do is fry your sliced bread on both sides in butter or margarine. Very good, but high in calories. It can be French fried, too.

Garlic toast. Mix 1/4 cup soft butter with 3/4 teaspoon garlic salt or a mashed sliver of garlic and spread on 6 slices toast. Good with soup or salad.

Ginger toast. Cream 1/4 cup butter, 1/2 cup brown sugar, 1 tablespoon minced candied ginger. Spread on toast and broil until bubbly. Cut into triangles.

Honey-pecan toast. Spread toast with butter, then with honey, sprinkle with crushed pecans, and broil 1 minute. Delicious with afternoon tea or a fruit-salad plate.

Lemon toast. Cream 1/4 cup butter with 1 teaspoon lemon juice, 1 teaspoon grated lemon rind. Spread on 6 slices bread toasted on underside and broil a few minutes. Serve with fish entrees. Add 2 tablespoons sugar and serve it as tea toast.

Maple-nut toast. Prepare bread as for honey-pecan toast, using maple syrup instead of honey. Or butter toast, spread with shaved maple sugar, add nuts, and broil.

Orange toast. Cream 1/4 cup butter, 2 tablespoons sugar or honey, and 1 tablespoon grated orange rind and spread on hot toast.

Rum-butter toast. For 6 slices toast, cream 1/4 cup butter, 1/2 cup confectioners' sugar, 1 tablespoon rum. Broil 1 minute. Cut in triangles.

SHORTCUTS USING CONVENIENCE FOODS

Potatoes

Sauerkraut. When baking sauerkraut, instead of grating raw potatoes, sprinkle a light layer of instant mashed potatoes between layers of sauerkraut and spareribs. This will absorb the liquid and retard the sharp flavor of the sauerkraut.

Rolls. For a quick dinner roll, with a special flavor, sift 1/2 cup instant potatoes with the dry ingredients into the liquid before mixing.

Soup. Instant Potato Soup. Sauté 1 teaspoon dehydrated onions in 2 tablespoons butter or butter substitute, season with salt and pepper according to taste. Add 1 scant tablespoon flour and 1/2 cup instant mashed potatoes. Serve with buttered croutons or plain. Before serving soup, garnish with chopped parsley or a dash of paprika. For a variation add 1 package dehydrated mushrooms or 1 can cream of mushroom soup.

Milk and Cheese

Milk and cheese are considered the perfect food; young and old require it. Cheese lovers will welcome the convenient tube or can dispensers for appetizers, snacks, garnishes on hors d'oeuvres. For a quick snack, use crackers, toast rounds, or squares. Squeeze from the tube in fancy designs, rosettes, or pipings.

Fill celery with your favorite cheese.

Spread cheese on bread, use a cookie cutter for fancy canapés. For a very attractive looking salad use a tomato, pear, or peach, fill the center with a cheese rosette. Make a cheese piping around a pear or pineapple for salad with cheese from a tube or can dispenser.

When serving croutons, for variety, decorate and garnish with your favorite cheese spread from a tube.

Cake Mixes

Quick Bar Cookies. Cut the liquid in half, add dates, chopped raisins, chocolate chips, coconut, cloves, or cinnamon.

If you want a sweeter dough when making shortcakes or upside down cakes, place fruit in a casserole baking dish, cake pan, or pie plate. Mix the cake mix according to directions, pour over the fruit, and bake following directions for upside down cake in regular recipes.

Tartar Sauce

To make a speedy tartar sauce take 1 cup sandwich spread, add 1 teaspoon catsup, 1 small onion grated or 1 tablespoon grated onion. 1/2 teaspoon Tabasco sauce is optional. Mix well. Serve with fish.

Pancake Mix

For a quick fritter batter, follow mixing directions on the package, cut the liquid to almost half, just enough to make a thick batter in which to dip fruit or eggplant for deep frying. Peel eggplant, cut into strips about 3 inches long, 1/4 to 1/2 inch wide. Dip into batter, coating eggplant completely. Fry on both sides until golden brown, about 3 minutes on each side. Drain on paper towels.

ATTRACTIVE GARNISH IDEAS

1. To make a lettuce cup, cut one head of lettuce in half, remove the core, hold under running water. The force of the water helps to separate the leaves. Fill lettuce cups with fruit salad, shredded cabbage salad, carrot salad. Fill lettuce cups for an attractive relish dish or tray with small pickles, stuffed olives, green or ripe olives, radishes, pickled onions.

2. Out of individual tartar sauce cups or servers? Cut 2 inches from the ends of a cucumber, scoop out the seeds to form a shell. Cut a scallop with a sharp knife on the ridge of the cucumber. Fill with tartar sauce or mayonnaise.

3. Run the sharp edge of fork prongs lengthwise on a peeled or unpeeled cucumber to give a ridge or scallop affect. Use as a garnish on a salad plate or slice thin when used in a tossed salad. As an added attraction to your cold-cut meat platter, cut cucumbers about 6/8 inch thick, slit halfway through the center. To make a twist, take one end of the slit, turn one end to the right, the other to the left, place on the platter.

4. To make orange or lemon twists, follow the same rules as for cucumber twists. Lemon twists add greatly to the appearance of fish. They can take the place of the usual lemon wedges served with fish.

5. Apple wedges filled with peanut butter add a creative and appealing look to a meat platter or a fruit and cheese plate. Use large red apples. Do not peel the apple, quarter, remove the seeds, cut in wedges about 1/4 inch thick. Spread with peanut butter, put together as a sandwich.

6. Cut a banana in half, spread with peanut butter, Put the other half of the banana on top. Cut in 1 or half inch pieces on a slant. This also enhances the salad plate or fruit plate on which it is served.

7. To prevent bananas from turning dark when using them as a base for a salad or as a garnish, drizzle lemon juice on the bananas or dip them in lemon juice. Use the sharp end of fork prongs lengthwise on peeled bananas to give a ridge effect.

8. Pineapple rings, rolled in colored sugar or chopped chives, fresh or dehydrated, make a very attractive base for salads or as a garnish for cold-cut trays or platters. Simply roll the edges in colored sugar or chives. Be sure to have the pineapple well drained or else the colored sugar will melt too fast.

9. To give a fern leaf effect to celery sticks, cut the celery in 3 to 4 inch lengths. With a sharp knife cut as closely as possible 1/4 inch slits down the side of the celery. Continue doing this on both sides of the celery stick until you've reached the bottom of the celery stick. Put in a large bowl of ice water at least 15 minutes until slits open up. Do not, however, keep the celery in water when storing in the refrigerator. Valuable vitamins are lost from vegetables if stored in water.

COMMON PIE TROUBLES AND HOW TO OVERCOME THEM

The tough crust. Too little shortening or too much water may cause your trouble. Handling the dough too much can make it tough. Rolling excess flour into it is bad. Roll pie crust on a floured pastry canvas with a stockinette-covered, lightly floured rolling pin or roll between two sheets of waxed paper. (Strangely enough, it is almost impossible to make a pastry-mix crust tough.)

The soaked crust. Get that pastry baked before it has a chance to soak. A constant temperature of 425° is best for most pies. Sometimes it helps to put part of the sugar and flour mixture for a fruit pie over the bottom crust before adding the fruit. With custard pies, avoid overbaking, which causes liquid to seep from the filling and soak the crust. Some cooks bake filling and pastry separately for custard pie, then slip the cooled filling into the baked crust.

The runny filling.　Pies including a variable amount of acid, such as lemon, chocolate, even butterscotch, need extra thickening, since the acid acts upon the starch to prevent its full effectiveness. Once in a while you may get an extra sour lemon in the pie you always make and find the filling thinner than you like it. In any cream filling, the cook should be sure to cook the starch mixture long enough to obtain the maximum thickening before adding eggs. After adding eggs, she should cook the mixture long enough to get the maximum thickening effect from them—usually about 3 minutes. Incidentally, sugar becomes liquid in the cooking, and a high proportion of sugar may tend to thin a filling.

The shrunken or bumpy crust.　Shrinkage is often caused by use of too much fat in the pastry; bumpiness by failure to get all the air out from under the crust before baking or failure to prick a pie shell evenly all over before it goes to the oven. Quick baking always helps in keeping the shape. The 425° oven is necessary for the single shell.

Juice that runs over.　Manufacturers have come up with all kinds of gadgets, including pie pans with extra rims and pie tape to seal the edges of a pie to prevent fruit fillings from boiling over. Thickening the filling before baking it in the pie prevents boiling over. One trick that helps is inserting short sticks of macaroni or straw sippers in openings in the upper crust or tucking in a paper cornucopia or china "pie bird" so that juices boil up into these and not out at the edges of the pie.

Seal pastry well at the edges; or top a fruit pie with lattice strips or an upper "floating" crust that doesn't meet the lower one but just sits on the filling. Then your pie won't boil over unless you've filled it entirely too full.

That weepy meringue.　To avoid this problem, spread the meringue so that it touches the edges of the pie all around and cool the baked fluff away from drafts, but not in the refrigerator. A common cause for weepiness is improper beating of the egg whites. Beat them at room temperature until they form soft peaks, then gradually beat in the sugar, 2 tablespoons for each white used, until it is all dissolved and the meringue is in stiff, shiny peaks. Too much sugar can make your pie cry.

Bake meringues 3 to 5 minutes at 400 to 425°. They'll be more tender and have less tendency to cry. They'll also cut more easily.

COOKIES
Margarine is a thoroughly satisfactory fat to use in making cookies. It has fine flavor and is economical. Flour for cookies almost invariably is the general-purpose type. It isn't necessary or even advisable to use cake flour unless the recipe specifically calls for it.

In many recipes, brown and white sugars can be used interchangeably, the brown giving a butterscotch kind of flavor to the cooky. When brown sugar is used, it should be free from lumps and packed tightly in the cup for measuring. Keep brown sugar moist by storing it in a tightly covered canister or in the breadbox. A slice of apple in the canister will keep the sugar soft or soften it if there are lumps. But take a rolling pin to any lumps, if you're in a hurry.

Shortcuts in Cooky Making
Here are some quick tricks in cooky making.

1. Mix the dough at night before you go to bed. Chill it overnight and do the baking the next day.

2. Instead of rolling and cutting cookies, try this trick occasionally: Shape little balls of the dough between the palms, place on cooky sheets, and flatten with a tumbler bottom moistened and dipped in sugar or covered with a damp cloth held by a rubber band. Some cookies can be flattened sufficiently by using the prongs of a fork vertically, then horizontally.

3. Instead of cutting rolled cookies with cutters, you can roll out a rectangle of dough, cut it in squares, diamonds, strips, or triangles, using a ruler for a guide and a pastry bag's jagger for pretty scalloped edges. This way you have no scraps to reroll and cut. You save time and work and avoid turning out any untender cookies, victims of too much rolling.

4. Almost any drop-cookie dough will also make bar cookies, which may be quicker. Just spread the dough quite thinly in a greased jelly-roll pan or other shallow baking pan. Be

sure the pans have sides, even if the dough seems stiff. Otherwise it may run over the edges and make a big mess out of your oven.

SOME COMMON CAUSES OF CAKE
FAILURES AND THEIR REMEDIES

The humped-in-the-middle split cake. This usually is the result of a too hot oven. Have the gas or electric company check your regulator. Too much flour in proportion to liquid also can do this. Did you sift the flour before measuring?

The heavy, solid layer at the bottom of a sponge cake. Oh, oh, you didn't beat those egg yolks enough! They should be thick and lemon colored, as the recipe says. Beat the sugar into them thoroughly, too.

The cake that falls. This could be the result of under-baking or using too large a pan for the size of the cake. Or too much shortening or sugar. Or too much or too little mixing of the batter.

The cake that's higher on one side. Maybe you spread it unevenly in the pan. Uneven oven heat can be the culprit. Or possibly your oven rack, or oven itself, isn't level. Most modern ranges are equipped with devices for adjusting the level if the kitchen floor is uneven.

The cake that runs over. There was too much batter for the pan.

The dry-textured cake. Too much flour, too little sugar, overbaking, or overbeating of egg whites—all can result in drying.

The coarse-textured cake. Overmixing or undermixing of the batter itself or of eggs or failure to cream butter and sugar sufficiently—these can produce coarse texture.

The tough cake. Usually this one has been overbeaten.

The angel food or sponge cake that falls out of the pan. Probably the cake needed more baking. Was the pan greased? It shouldn't have been! However, it is all right to grease an angel food pan and use it for coffee cake. A good sudsy washing will remove every trace of fat before the next angel food is baked. Watery egg whites can result in a cake that falls from the pan.

Good Technique Counts in Making Cakes

The first step in cakemaking is assembling ingredients. In any good kitchen all ingredients are assembled on a tray before the mixing begins. The flour is always sifted once before measuring (onto a sheet of waxed paper). Then it is spooned lightly into the cup and leveled off with a spatula. Cake flour is lighter in texture than general-purpose flour. Use cake flour if the recipe directs you to or sift general-purpose flour several times, measure, and take out a tablespoonful. If you use self-rising flour, omit salt and baking powder.

Break eggs right out of the refrigerator, but let them warm to room temperature before beating, as they'll give you more volume. Use the best eggs for flavor and volume. Avoid the common mistake of breaking an egg right into the bowl when your mixer is running. You may get a poor flavored egg, and then your batter is lost. Or you might let some shell drop into the batter. Break each egg into a cup or sauce dish first.

Measure dry ingredients in cups that can be leveled off at the top, and measure liquids in glass measures designed for liquids, with extra space at the top above the measured markings. Sift the dry ingredients together several times before adding them to the batter.

Use shortening if your recipe calls for shortening, butter if it specifies butter. Special formulas and special techniques have been developed for the shortening cakes. Don't think you'll improve them with butter.

Use the correct pan size and shape. Avoid the dented, battered pan. Good baking equipment is not expensive. If you bake in glass, reduce the temperature 25°. Have pans greased and lined with waxed paper before you begin to mix. Fill pans not more than two thirds full and smooth the batter in the pans. If you use odd-shaped pans, fill not more than half full.

Have the oven preheated, bake for the proper length of time, and be certain to cool your cake on a rack. Cool it 5 minutes in the pan, then loosen at the sides and turn out, so that air can circulate around the cake and prevent a soggy crust. Angel, sponge, and chiffon cakes are not cooled this way, of course. They're exceptions.

How Do You Tell When a Cake is Done?

You can use a cake tester or a toothpick, but if the cake has shrunk away from the sides of the pan and if the surface springs back when you press it with your forefinger, the cake should be done. A good recipe and an accurate oven will usually bake the cake done for you in the time specified. But always make a test to be certain.

Little Tricks that Help

For even-sized layers weigh the batter into prepared pans by scales or divide by spoonfuls for the same amount in each pan.

If you want to cut squares, use a ruler and toothpicks to mark off even spaces along the sides of your cake. When you divide an angel or sponge cake into layers, stick toothpicks in the sides to guide your knife or circle the cake at the proper intervals with No. 50 thread, then gently pull the thread tight to cut the cake into even layers.

Cream the sugar and shortening very, very fast. This step is important, and it is almost impossible to overbeat at this stage.

Beat egg yolks long and vigorously for sponge cake. The most common cause of failure in this type of cake is under-beating those yolks. They'll make a heavy layer at the bottom of the cake if they're not sufficiently beaten.

Beat egg whites until they stand in peaks, but be careful not to overbeat them, except in the case of a chiffon cake, when overbeaten whites are actually required. Stir beaten egg whites into batter quickly. Speed is more important than gentleness.

Where Do You Keep a Filled and Frosted Cake?

Keep it in the refrigerator if the filling or frosting is made with eggs. Otherwise a covered cake plate or the bread-box is fine.

YEAST BREADS

Ingredients in Addition to Yeast

Flour. Enriched white flour is the principal ingredient of most yeast breads. All-purpose flour is needed because of its gluten, a protein that is elastic and stretches to accommodate the gas bubbles formed by the yeast. Cake flour, which is much weaker in gluten, is not suitable. Self-rising flour does not produce a good yeast bread, either, as a rule. If you use it, be sure to follow a recipe especially adapted for it.

Whole wheat, rye, soy, and buckwheat flours sometimes are used in yeast breads, usually in combination with white flour, since any of them alone produces a rather heavy, compact loaf. Cornmeal, rolled oats, and bran are other cereal ingredients now and then employed in fairly small quantities to change the flavor and texture of yeast breads.

Sugar, Salt. It takes very little of either to make good yeast dough. Sugar helps the yeast to work, but a little sugar is all it takes—frequently only one tablespoon to a batch of dough. Salt helps control the action of yeast, and while it is possible to make a salt-free yeast bread, dough without salt rises rapidly and must be watched closely.

Water versus Milk. Breads made with milk are more nutritious, keep better, have a more velvety texture. Those made with water have a wheatier flavor and crisper crust. Take your choice or use half of one, half of the other. Sometimes fruit juice is used as part of the liquid for the flavor it produces.

Any liquid should be warm, about 110°, for active dry yeast or lukewarm, about 85°, for compressed yeast. Milk must be scalded and then cooled (evaporated milk may be used without scalding, likewise reconstituted dry milk).

Shortening. Use butter, vegetable or lard shortening, oil, or margarine. Most yeast breads require a very small amount, but shortening does help form an elastic structure in rising dough and increases tenderness.

Eggs. Eggs are used in coffee cakes and rolls quite frequently and in the sweeter loaves of bread. They tend to give a more cake-like texture, promote browning of the crust, and, of course, add nutritive qualities to the bread. Eggs as well as other ingredients of bread should be at room temperature when used in order not to slow the action of the yeast.

Refrigerator Doughs and Frozen Doughs

When a dough is richer than usual in fat and sugar, it will keep for as long as four or five days in the refrigerator, to be used as needed for rolls and coffee cake. Yeast dough may be frozen, but it is better to freeze the baked bread or rolls.

Temperature for Mixing Yeast Doughs and Letting Them Rise

Yeast is a plant that enjoys a cozy warm temperature, but it is easily killed when it becomes too hot. Slay your yeast in the oven, not before it has had time to leaven your dough.

Active dry yeast dissolves best in water at a temperature described as warm. Warm is about 105 to 110°. Compressed yeast is better off at the old familiar lukewarm temperature of 85 to 90°, a point at which water feels neither warm nor cool to your fingers. Compressed yeast liquifies with sugar, but active dry yeast performs most efficiently when dissolved in warm water.

Rising temperatures should be between 82° and 85°. This is sometimes a difficult temperature to achieve in winter. One good method is to set the bowl of rising dough into a deep pan of warm water. Dough may be placed near a radiator or operating burner on a range, but beware of putting it on the radiator or warm burner. It may get too warm.

How to Knead Yeast Doughs

"Kneading" means blending the dough by manipulating it quickly with the hands. Its purpose is to stretch the dough until it becomes smooth, elastic, and no longer sticky. About 8 to 10 minutes of kneading is usually sufficient. Here is the correct method to use:

Working quickly, flatten the dough slightly on a lightly floured board with the hands. With the fingers, fold the dough over on itself toward you. Push the dough away from you with your palms, then grasp the dough with both hands and turn it a quarter of a way around on the board or pastry cloth. Repeat this manipulation, working firmly with a rocking motion.

Rising of Yeast Doughs

Grease the bowl containing the dough and grease the top of the dough to prevent it from becoming crusty. Cover the bowl with a towel to keep it warm. When the weather is cold, warm the bowl slightly before adding the ball of dough. Set the bowl in a warm place (80 to 85°) away from drafts. It may be an unlighted oven, a closed cupboard, or a table set away from doors and windows. Let the dough rise until twice its original volume. The time can vary greatly, depending on flour used, other ingredients, and temperature, so check the size of the dough occasionally. If in doubt about whether it has risen sufficiently, plunge a finger deeply into the center of the dough, remove it at once. If indentation remains, the dough probably has doubled in bulk. It may take from 1 to 1 1/2 hours to rise the first time. The second rising takes somewhat shorter time.

How to Shape Loaves

With the hands, press the dough for one loaf into an oblong about 9 by 8 inches. Fold each end of the oblong to the center, pressing down firmly. Pinch together the center fold and each end of dough to seal tightly. Place loaf, sealed side down, in greased bread pan. Do not force dough to all corners of your pan; on rising and during baking it will expand sufficiently to fill the pan and give a nicely rounded loaf.

A Caution about Rising Time

"Let rise until light" or "Let rise until doubled in bulk" are better guides than a specified time, since there are many variable factors affecting time, including the amount of yeast used. Stollen and other breads rich in shortening, sugar, or eggs, and containing fruit take longer to rise than plainer breads. (They take longer to bake, too.)

Note: At high altitudes, bread rises faster than usual.

Food Saving Checklist

1. Day-old baked breads, rolls, and cakes are usually marked down but are as fresh as if you'd bought them yesterday and stored them at home. If you have ample freezing space, buy enough of these marked down baked goods for 1 to 2 weeks at a time.

2. Storing bread in the refrigerator or freezer extends the freshness, and you can drastically cut down on the amount that is wasted by staleness or mold.

3. Use unused foods wisely. Small quantities of vegetables, for example, can be used in soups or combined with other vegetables as a new, creative dish.

4. Store foods properly. When you return home from the supermarket and also after meals, put food away quickly to avoid spoilage and waste. This is especially important for perishable items.

5. Imitation sour cream is less expensive than real sour cream. When used in hot dishes such as stroganoff and lasagna, you cannot tell the difference.

6. Dips made from sour cream are just as tasty as pre-packaged dips—and about half the price for twice the amount.

7. Plan for snacks. Homemade snacks such as cookies, fruit drinks, and milk-based drinks are usually less expensive than store-bought snacks and are most always more nutritious.

8. Bacon is an extra flavor as well as a meat choice. A few slices diced, cooked, and stirred into scrambled eggs stretch a little a long way. The drippings make ideal seasoners for vegetables and salads.

9. Experiment with spices and seasonings. Garlic, mustard, Worcestershire sauce, chili, catsup, and horseradish are relatively low in cost and quick to use. Using a wide range of seasonings and flavors that you like adds variety at minimal cost, encourages consumption of fruits and vegetables, increases the use of foods that are low in calories, and reduces the need for sauces that are too costly.

10. Make oven heat do double or triple duty. For example, bake a stew along with a roast or a big squash in the shell to peel or cut up and glaze for another meal or cook your whole meal in the oven at one time. By using your oven for double duty, you will decrease your gas or electric bill.

11. Macaroni, noodles, and dried beans are excellent for a meatless meal.

12. Purchase staples such as flour, sugar, and cornmeal only in large amounts, if possible. The majority of food products cost less if you purchase them in bulk.

13. Check sales for two, three, four, or five of the same items for a certain price. They usually mean big savings if the foods are ones your family likes.

14. Use bouillon cubes or envelopes of instant broth in lieu of canned broth, which costs more.

15. Bake your own cakes instead of purchasing them. It is about 75 percent cheaper.

16. Save liquid from cooked and canned fruits and vegetables. Store in refrigerator and use for soups, stews, casseroles, for meat cooking, or in lieu of water in gelatin desserts.

17. Refrigerate eggs promptly at home, large ends up, to help maintain quality. Variations in temperature while the eggs are stored cause egg whites to become thin.

18. Cool leftover meat, broth, and gravies quickly and store, well covered, in the refrigerator. Use within 1 to 3 days after cooking.

19. Use in meals some of the less expensive sources of protein such as dry beans, peas, and lentils, peanut butter, eggs, and cheese.

20. Use all vegetable scraps for soup stock. Do not throw them away.

Use of Seasonings

Bay Leaves.   Greeks used bay leaves to crown their victorious heroes. A wise cook will use bay leaves as a crowning victory to stews, beef roasts, and chicken soup. Cook two or three leaves, depending on size with kidney, tongue, or heart. When cooking vegetable soup or chowders, add one or two bay leaves. Remove bay leaf before serving. Don't forget to include bay leaves when preparing your pickling syrup. Add bay leaves to tomatoes while cooking for tomato juice. As a variation, bay leaves also give added flavor to tomato stew.

Parsley.   Fresh, dried, or frozen. Add to stews, vegetable soups. Sprinkle over potato salad, macaroni, and cottage cheese for color effect. Add to salads. Use fresh as a garnish on meat platters, salads, relish dishes.

Caraway Seed.   Excellent as additional flavor to sauerkraut. Add to rye bread according to taste. For something different on a cracker or as a filling for canapes, add caraway seed to cream cheese, mix well. When mixing corn bread, add a small amount of caraway seeds. A decidedly different twist to the lowly corn bread.

Celery Seed.   Mix with cream sauces for vegetables. Add to salad dressings. Add to cabbage, carrots, and turnips for a variation. Caution: add a small amount, vegetable flavor should predominate.

Chili Powder.   Chili powder does wonders to a meat loaf, hamburgers, meat sauces. Tired of the same taste when drinking tomato juice? Next time add a small sprinkle to your chilled tomato juice. Chili powder added according to taste makes chili and beans the favorite of young and old.

Oregano.   A must when preparing sauces for pizza and spaghetti. When making tomato stew, a small pinch will go a long way to perk up this nutritious dish.

Mint.   Use fresh mint as garnish for salads and meat and cheese platters. Adds a refreshing flavor to cool drinks. When boiling apple mint jelly, add to apple juice, remove from jelly before bottling. Excellent served with lamb and pork.

Sage.   Add a pinch to your cream sauce when preparing chicken à la king. Add to rice and bread dressing used in stuffed fowl, chops, veal breasts, standing ribs, crown roasts.

Rub outside of turkey and fowl with sage powder before roasting. To improve flavor in pork, sprinkle on top slightly before roasting.

Cinnamon. Cinnamon added to apples for sauce, besides giving off a pungent odor, adds greatly to the flavor. Add cinnamon to baked apples, apple crisp, strained apple sauce, baked rice pudding. Sprinkle on top of cider when serving hot cider. Use a cinnamon-sugar mixture on French toast, hot cooked cereal, cinnamon toast. Here are some other foods in which cinnamon can be used:

Coffee cake topping	Apple pie
Cinnamon rolls	Mock apple pie
Sugar cookie topping	Pumpkin pie
Gingerbread topping	Rhubarb pie
Cornbread topping	Rhubarb sauce

Sprinkle cinnamon on hot burner if milk has accidentally boiled over. The cinnamon will not harm the burner; as it burns a pungent odor will fill the room.

Stick Cinnamon. Use in pickling syrup for apple rings, pears, peaches.

Cloves. Use sparingly, unless a strong clove taste is desired. When baking ham, stud with whole cloves before baking. Whole cloves: use in making pickling syrup. Ground cloves: use in ginger cookies, pumpkin pie, gingerbread, nut breads, and apple-plum butter. Add a whole clove to apples when making apple juice. Before broiling pears or peaches, fill with brown sugar and butter, sprinkle cloves over the top. When baking acorn squash, fill centers with brown sugar and butter and sprinkle with cloves. Bake squash upside down until done, before putting in the sugar and butter mixture. Squash will be moist if a little water is added to the pan while baking.

Basil. Excellent as a seasoning with vegetables. Also is used as a seasoning on lamb roast.

Onions. Fresh, frozen, dehydrated, onion salt. Onion salt can be a very good substitute for raw onions. People who cannot digest fresh, frozen, or dehydrated onions have found that they can enjoy the flavor of onion when a substitute is used. Onions can be used effectively with meats, vegetables, and salads. Onions should be used sparingly. They are meant to add flavor not predominate, unless they are used as a vegetable or garnish, for example, as an accompaniment on a relish dish or tossed salad. Onions if used moderately help bring out the flavor of meats and salads. Sauté onions in butter or butter substitute before using as a seasoning—this helps to produce a more delicate flavor. To avoid shedding useless tears when peeling an onion, hold under cold running water, peel off outer skin.

If a recipe calls for a small amount of onion, chop or slice the rest of the onion and freeze it. Use small plastic sandwich bags. In this way you'll have the right amount the next time you need onions. They will retain their true flavor indefinitely.

Chives.   Fresh, frozen, dehydrated. If an onion flavor is desired, a good substitute available the whole year is chives. Chives give additional flavor to salads, scrambled eggs, cream sauces, salad dressings, chip dips, and vegetables. Just before serving cottage cheese, add fresh chives. They will retain their crispness and fresh green color. Add to cream cheese and serve shaped into balls, on toothpicks, with crackers and tomato juice. Sprinkle on top of chowders and cream soups just before serving. Sprinkle on top of croutons while butter is still hot. They will adhere to butter and give added flavor to soups. Dehydrated chives can be used in the same way as fresh or frozen. Dehydrated chives and onions are time-savers, convenient, economical, easy to use. Keep in airtight containers at all times to retain flavor.

Garlic.   Fresh or dried. The flavor of roast beef can be enhanced by sprinkling minced garlic on top of the roast before roasting. Use sparingly. Garlic salt used sparingly will also improve the flavor of other meats. Rub a wooden salad bowl or mixing bowl with a fresh bud of garlic before mixing tossed salads. To give additional flavor to casserole foods, rub the casserole with a garlic bud. The flavor will gradually be absorbed by the food as it heats. Mince garlic very fine, sauté in butter until golden brown, add to sauces. Used in preparing spaghetti, meat balls, and pizza, ravioli, or rice dishes, using a tomato sauce. Mash a small bud of garlic and add to cheddar cheese for an unusual spread on canapés and crackers.

Garlic salt, onion salt, and dried or dehydrated chives are convenient when you want to whip up a quick snack or hot bread for company dinner. Slice a loaf of French or Vienna bread into 1/4 inch slices. Butter one side, sprinkle salt or chives on one side, continue until all slices are used. Put into loaf shape, wrap in foil wrap. Heat oven at 325°. Heat the bread about 20 to 30 minutes.

Cheeses and Wines

**Some Common Cheeses
and How to Use Them**

American-made Cheddar Cheese.   Commonly called simply "American cheese," this can be mild or sharp, pale yellow to deep orange, process or natural. Cheese lovers want it aged and sharp. The process Americans melt readily, so are the usual choice for cooking. This is the cheese used for rabbits, sauces, sandwiches, casseroles, the general handyman among cheese, the every-purpose kind.

Apple.   A hard, sharp-flavored, apple-shaped, smoked cheese of Italian origin. Eaten as cheese, not much used in cooking.

Asiago.   A hard cheese of granular texture and piquant flavor. Italian in origin, it is eaten as table cheese or used grated.

Bel Paese.   An Italian table and dessert cheese, mild flavored, of soft, spongy texture.

Blue and bleu.   The former is American blue-mold cheese, the latter, French. Both are Roquefort types, sharp in flavor, much used in appetizers, salad dressings, and as dessert. There is also a Danish blue cheese of excellent quality and much of that is consumed in the United States.

Brick.   An American semi-hard cheese that comes in brick shape, with many tiny round holes. The flavor is a little like Swiss, a little like Limburger. Good eaten plain, in sandwiches, or cut into julienne strips for mixed green salads.

Brie.   A French soft dessert cheese, also made in Canada and the United States. It resembles Camembert in size, shape, texture, and in that it has the same type of rind, but it is sharper in flavor. With fresh apples, pears, or grapes and toasted crackers, a superlative dessert.

Caciocavallo. This is often called "horse cheese," because, it is said, the imprint of a horse's head appeared on the original cheese as a trademark. Shaped like a beet or a tenpin, this hard, smoked Italian cheese is used most frequently, in grated form, as a seasoning.

Camembert. Soft, mold-ripened cheese of French origin with a gray-white rind and creamy interior. A favorite dessert cheese. Much like Brie and served frequently with fruit as well as crackers. A great delicacy.

Cheddar. One of the oldest and most popular of English cheeses. It is a hard cheese, mild to sharp. This cheese is sometimes known as "American" or "American Cheddar." The name was derived from the village of Cheddar in Somersetshire, England. Hundreds of uses in cooking and a favorite table and dessert cheese.

Cheshire. Like Cheddar, but stronger and sharper, and usually colored deep yellow. It is made in huge 50- to 70-pound cylinders. Cheshire County, England, is its home. One of the oldest and most popular of English cheeses.

Club cheese. This term applies to a large variety of soft, blended, natural cheeses, usually Cheddar types, which come in crocks or pots or other containers and are used as spreads. They often are highly seasoned with condiments, wine, or smoke flavor.

Cottage. Soft, white, tender curds, an unripened cheese made of skimmed milk. Cream may be added later. Bland in flavor and highly prized for table use. Often seasoned with onion or chives and served as an appetizer. Makes excellent salads, cheese cake.

Cream. A soft, buttery, smooth white cheese eaten fresh. It is highly popular as a spread and chief ingredient in homemade cheese mixes and dips. Used in salads, as dessert with fruit, and in desserts such as rich cheese cakes.

Daisy®. This is a trade name for a disc-shaped American Cheddar cheese, weighing about 20 pounds, that may be cut in wedges for sale to the consumer.

Edam.   A hard, rather rubbery-textured Dutch cheese with a nutty flavor. Comes in "cannon ball" shape. Eaten as a table cheese and sometimes as dessert. There's a "baby" Edam, slightly smaller. Coated with a red rind.

Gammelost.   A hard, golden brown, strong-flavored Norwegian cheese, a smorgasbord type.

Gjetost.   Goat's milk cheese. Hard, very dark brown, granular, and sweetish in flavor. Norwegian, and found on the smorgasbord.

Gorgonzola.   This is the Italian version of Roquefort, blue or bleu. A blue-mold cheese, crumbly textured, used in salads, as dessert, in spreads.

Gouda.   A semi-hard cheese from Holland, similar to Edam and coated with a red rind. Looks like Edam, but the ball is flattened.

Gruyere.   A semi-hard, process Swiss. Melts more easily than Swiss. The prime ingredient of Swiss fondue and a favorite dessert cheese with toasted crackers. The flavor is nutty.

Hand.   Small, sour-milk cheese of strong flavor and odor. Too smelly to be generally popular.

Herkimer.   Herkimer County, New York, is famous for a very sharp uncolored Cheddar. An excellent cheese for table or dessert use. Much New York Cheddar is of this type.

Jack or Monterey Jack.   This isn't so well known outside of California, where it is made. It's a semi-hard, smooth, mild cheese, used for sandwiches and as table cheese, and to some extent in cooking.

Leyden.   A Dutch cheese much like Edam, but containing caraway seeds. Popular for table use and good on a tray of assorted cheeses.

Liederkranz®. This is an American cheese made exclusively by one manufacturer. A relative of Limburger, but less pungent, it is soft and smelly, but quite mild in flavor. Good with crackers. Used somewhat in dips and spreads, often in combination with cream cheese. Not a bad dessert cheese. Comes in a foil-wrapped 4-ounce cake.

Limburger. A larger, stronger, smellier cheese than Liederkranz. Originally Belgian, it is made domestically to a considerable extent. Used in sandwiches and with crackers. Limburger also is processed.

Longhorn. This is just good old American Cheddar shaped in a cylinder about 5 inches in diameter and 12 to 13 inches long. Wrapped in cheesecloth.

Mozzarella. This is the Italian favorite for pizza and some macaroni and spaghetti dishes. It also can be crumbed and fried. Mozzarella is a fresh, unsalted, soft, bland cheese that comes in small egg shapes or twists. It sometimes is salted and smoked.

Muenster. A semi-soft cheese of German origin, creamy white inside. Used for sandwiches and on cheese trays. The flavor is mild and mellow.

Mysost. This is a buttery-textured, light-brown, mild Scandinavian cheese, often found on the smorgasbord. It isn't often served except as table cheese.

Neufchâtel. This is a French cheese of smooth, soft texture, much like cream cheese. It is popular for salads, canapés, sandwiches, table, and dessert use.

Oka. The Canadian Port du Salut, made by Trappist monks, also known as Trappist cheese. It comes in a 1- or 5-pound cake, russet on the outside, semi-soft and creamy yellow within. It is mildly odoriferous, but well liked in general. Used on the cheese tray, with pie, as a dessert cheese.

Parmesan. The familiar form is grated. It is an aged, hard cheese, made in 50- to 60-pound cylinders, with a dark-green surface. Popular sprinkled on all kinds of Italian specialties, especially spaghetti and minestrone. Makes a fine casserole topping.

Pineapple. This is a hard American Cheddar cheese, shaped like a pineapple because of the method of drying in a coarse-meshed net. It is rubbed with linseed oil and shellacked on the outside.

Pont l'Eveque. So similar to Brie that only connoisseurs would be able to distinguish between them. French, and a dessert cheese.

Port du Salut. The cheese made by Trappist monks in France and Canada. See Oka.

Primost. The Scandinavian cheese also known as Mysost. Unripened, made from whey, it is soft, light brown, mild in flavor, and seldom eaten except as a table cheese.

Process. This term refers to natural cheeses that have been ground, blended with an emulsifying agent, melted, and pasteurized. Process cheeses melt more easily than natural cheeses and can be standardized in quality. They also keep better. They are fine for cooking, spreads, and sandwiches; however, most cheese lovers prefer the natural cheeses as table cheese. About a third of our natural cheeses end up pasteurized and processed, many of them with added flavoring agents—bacon, ham, pimiento, chives, possibly smoke flavor, and garlic.

Provolone. An Italian pear-shaped hard cheese that is smoked and has a rather sharp flavor. It is a "slicing" cheese, served as such.

Ricotta. Fresh, moist unsalted Italian cheese similar to our cottage cheese.

Romano. In Italy it is made of sheep's milk, domestically, of cow's milk. This is a hard, grating cheese of sharp, tangy flavor. Used in many Italian-type dishes and for sprinkling over casseroles and into soup.

Roquefort. The original French blue-veined cheese, made from sheep's milk (blue, bleu, Gorgonzola, and Stilton, its imitators from other lands, are cow's milk cheeses) and ripened in the famous caves near Roquefort, France. A dessert cheese, also widely used in spreads, dips, salad dressings, on steaks.

Samsoe. A popular Danish cheese, mild and creamy,

with a nutty flavor. It is characterized by small holes. Used for sandwiches and in cooking.

Sapsago. What the moon is made of—green cheese! This is a hard Swiss cheese for grating. The color comes from a clover-like plant used as flavoring. Made of sour milk, buttermilk, and whey.

Scamorze or Scamozza. An Italian fresh, pear-shaped cheese that melts with a characteristic stringiness. Used for pizza, casseroles. Resembles Mozzarella.

Stilton. The English blue-mold cheese that has been made since the mideighteenth century. It is sharp flavored and usually is aged 2 years before it is eaten. Served as dessert cheese, with salads, and in all the ways liked for Roquefort, blue, bleu, and Gorgonzola.

Swiss. The cheese with the "eyes" produced by gas in the curing. A favorite sandwich, salad, and cheese-tray cheese, of sweetish, nutty flavor. Emmenthaler is the true Swiss cheese, but huge quantities of "Swiss" are made in this country.

CHEESE AND WINE COMBINATIONS

Brie. Red table wines. Sparkling wines.

Camembert. Red or white table wines or any of the sparkling or dessert wines.

Cheddar. Red table wines (the same are served with American cheese).

Edam and Gouda. Red table wines or dessert wines when the cheese is served as part of a dessert cheese tray.

Gruyere. White table wines, particularly the Swiss.

Gorgonzola. Red table wines. Try a Burgundy, Chianti, or even a dry Sherry.

Monterey Jack. Red table wines, although the lighter red wines and rosés are best.

Note: Persons on low-cholesterol diets should seek the advice of their physicians as to their intake of cheese.

Dessert wines are best served at cool room temperature.

Despite the number of "rules" given for the service of specific cheeses with wines, modernists like to serve the cheese of their choice with their favorite wines, regardless of whether they "go together" or not.

When serving cheese and wine for dessert, select a variety of cheese with different flavors and textures—some soft, some hard, some mild, some sharp. With crisp crackers or bread, colorful grapes, yellow or red apples, some fresh pears, and a bottle of wine—red or white table wines, or even a sparkling wine—the dessert cheese tray makes a dramatic finale for any meal.

Checklist for Proper Menu Planning

For convenience in planning, I have classified the most common everyday foods into eleven groups in the following lists, and the number of servings needed daily to provide an adequate diet is indicated. Although the lists are not complete, they can be used in placing most foods in their proper group. Miscellaneous items such as coffee and tea, seasonings and flavorings, and baking powder and soda are not included in the eleven groups.

LEAFY, GREEN, AND YELLOW VEGETABLES
(Fresh, Canned, Frozen)
Plan to use: 1 or more servings daily

Asparagus, green	Okra
Beans, lima	Peas
Beans, snap, green	Peppers, green
Broccoli	Pumpkin
Brussels sprouts	Spinach
Cabbage, green	Squash, winter yellow
Carrots	Turnip greens
Kale	Wild greens
Mustard greens	Other greens, including salad greens

CITRUS FRUIT, TOMATOES
(Fresh, Canned, Frozen)
Plan to use: 1 or more servings daily

Grapefruit	Oranges
Lemons	Tangerines
Limes	Tomatoes and Tomato products

The following foods are also good sources of Vitamin C and may be used to supplement citrus fruit and tomatoes; raw green cabbage, salad greens, raw green peppers, raw turnips, raw strawberries, raw pineapple, cantaloupe (musk-melon).

POTATOES, SWEET POTATOES
(Fresh, Canned)
Plan to use: 1 or more servings daily
Potatoes   Sweet Potatoes

OTHER VEGETABLES AND FRUITS
(Fresh, Canned, Frozen, Dried)
Plan to use: 1 or more servings daily or additional servings of leafy, green or yeallow vegetables

Apples	Cherries	Grapes	Plums
Apricots	Corn, Sweet	Melons	Prunes
Bananas	Cranberries	Onions	Radishes
Beets	Cucumbers	Parsnips	Raisins
Berries	Currants	Peaches	Summer Squash
Cauliflower	Dates	Pears	Turnips
Celery	Figs	Pineapple	Watermelons

MILK, CHEESE, ICE CREAM
Plan to use daily the following amounts of milk or its equivalent. The quantities include milk used both for drinking and for cooking. Adults: 2 or more cups. The group includes:

Milk, fluid	Milk, condensed
Milk, skim	Buttermilk
Milk, dry, whole	Cheese
Milk, dry, nonfat	Ice Cream
Milk, evaporated	

MEAT, POULTRY, FISH
(Fresh, Canned, Cured, Frozen, Dried)
Plan to use: One or more servings daily (include liver or other variety meats once a week, if possible). Additional servings of eggs may be used in place of meat on occasion.

Beef	Tongue
Lamb	Sweetbreads
Mutton	Chicken
Pork (except bacon and fat back)	Duck
	Goose
Veal	Turkey
Liver	Fish, all kinds

EGGS
Plan to use: 3 to 5 a week or additional servings of meat, poultry, fish.

DRY BEANS AND PEAS, NUTS
Plan to use: 1 or more servings a week

Dry Beans (all kinds)	Soya flour and grits
Dry Peas	Peanuts
Lentils	Peanut Butter
Soybeans	Nuts, all kinds

FLOUR, CEREALS, BAKED GOODS
Plan to use: Some enriched whole-grain, or restored cereals or cereal products daily, others as needed for satisfying meals.

Flour, enriched or whole grain, all types	Bread, enriched or whole grain, all kinds	Cookies
Cooked cereals	Rolls	Crackers
Ready-to-eat cereals	Cakes	Pies

FATS AND OILS
Plan to use: Some butter or fortified margarine daily; other fats as needed in cooking.

Butter	Bacon
Margarine	Salt Pork
Mayonnaise	Shortening
Salad Dressing	Suet
Salad Oil	Drippings

SUGAR, SYRUPS, PRESERVES
Plan to use: As needed for food energy and flavor in meals.

Sugar (cane or beet)	Jams
Sugar, Brown	Jellies
Molasses	Preserves
Syrups	Candies
Honey	

With the basic needs defined in terms of nutrients and the foods that supply them, the next step is to plan to use these foods in attractive and satisfying meals.

USE OF LEFT-OVERS. In spite of careful planning, the problem of left-overs may arise. When foods have been left over, try to fit them into other meals as soon as possible. Even though left-overs lose some food value during storage and re-heating, they usually retain enough to make them worth using.

The suggestions on the list below illustrate some of the kinds of dishes in which left-overs can be used.

SUGGESTIONS FOR USE OF LEFTOVERS

Cooked Meats	Cooked Potatoes	Cooked Vegetables
Croquettes	Creamed	Soup
Meat Pie	Fried	Meat Pie
Hash	Potato Cakes	Stew
Casserole dishes	Stuffed	Stuffed Peppers
Sandwich	Baked	Salads
fillings	Meat Pie	
Salads	Stew	
	Chowder	
	Hash	

Cooked Cereals	Bread, Cakes	Eggs
Fried	Bread, dry crumbs	Egg yolks
Meat Loaf	Brown Betty	Cakes
Rice, with	Breaded chops	Pie Fillings
tomatoes		Salad Dressing
Croquettes		
Fondue		

Milk	Macaroni	Soft Crumbs
Sour Milk	Noodles	Meat Loaf
Cakes	Tomatoes	Stuffing
Cookies	Cheese	Cake or Cookies
Muffins	Meat Sauce	Brown Betty
Cottage	Tunafish	Ice-box Cake
Cheese		

Egg Whites	Sour Cream	Cooked Eggs
Meringue	Cakes	Deviled
Cake	Cookies	Creamed
Puddings	Salad Dressing	Salads
	Swiss Steak	Sandwich
		fillings

SAMPLE MENUS FOR 2 DAYS SHOWING HOW

FOOD GROUP	BREAKFAST	DINNER	LUNCH OR SUPPER
Leafy, green and yellow vegetable		Broccoli	Green Lettuce
Citrus fruit, tomatoes	Grapefruit Juice		Tomato
Potatoes, sweet-potatoes		Sweet-Potatoes	
Other vege-tables and fruit		Celery Sticks Radishes Apples in Pie	Peaches
Milk, cheese, ice cream	Milk		Milk
Meat, poultry fish		Roast Shoulder of Pork	
Eggs	Scrambled Eggs		
Dry beans and peas, nuts			Baked Lima Beans
Flour, cereal, baked goods	Toast Wheat cereal	Rolls Apple Pie	Raisin Bread Oatmeal cookies
Fats, oils,(a)	Butter or Margarine	B or M	B or M Salad Dress.
Sugar, syrups, preserves(b)	Jam		

(a) Other fat used in cooking
(b) Other sugar used in cooking and beverages

FOODS FROM 11 GROUPS CAN BE USED

BREAKFAST	DINNER	LUNCH OR SUPPER
	Green cabbage (salad) Carrots	Green Asparagus
Tomato Juice	Orange Scalloped potatoes	
	Prunes (salad)	Whipped gelatin with bananas
	Meat Loaf	Ham ala King on Toast
		Eggs in Ham ala King
	Nuts (done in salad)	
Toast Scrapple	Bread Butterscotch pudding	Rolls
B or M	B or M Gravy	B or M
Syrup		Jelly

PLANNING FOR NUTRITION

It is a well known fact that most of us do not consume the daily requirements of vitamins for proper body function and growth. In some cases, this deficiency is countered by the intake of vitamin pills; in others, by the eating of specific foods high in vitamin content. However, prolonged absence of the daily requirements of any particular nutrient will result in harmful effects in the body itself and in the function of the senses and capabilities of the person. In an effort to identify these characteristics and the vitamin which may be lacking in particular cases, a list is printed below which associates the signs of poor health that may accompany an insufficient intake of protective food in the diet.

<u>Vitamin A</u>–	A dry, scaly or "goose pimple" skin, ingrown hair, low resistance to infection, diarrhea, sensitivity of eyes to bright light, night blindness.
<u>Vitamin B$_1$</u>	(thiamin chloride)—Lassitude, no energy for work, poor appetite, constipation, nervousness and irritability, poor judgment, sleeplessness, neuralgia.
<u>Vitamin C</u>–	(ascorbic acid)—Lassitude, no energy for work, skin hemorrhages, spongy bleeding gums, low resistance to infection, slowly healing wounds, tooth disorders.
<u>Vitamin D</u>–	Poor teeth, crooked bones, rickets.
<u>Vitamin B$_2$</u>	(Riboflavin)—Burning itching eyes sensitive to light, blackheads and "whiteheads," oily skin, sore lips with cracks at corners.
<u>Niacin</u>	(formerly known as nicotinic acid)—Sore mouth and tongue, burning of throat, rough, chapped skin particularly in winter, sleeplessness, indigestion, nervousness, constipation, loss in weight.
<u>Calcium</u>–	Tooth cavities, poorly developed bones and teeth, muscle soreness.
<u>Iron</u>–	Lassitude and fatigue, general weakness, nutritional anemia, mental dullness.
<u>Iodine</u>–	Lassitude and fatigue, simple goiter.
<u>Protein</u>	Tiredness, general weakness, anemia, loss of weight, edema.

PRINCIPAL SOURCES OF ENERGY FOODS

Starches	Sugars	Fats
Breads	Sugar	Butter
Crackers	Molasses	Cream
Rice	Honey	Lard
Breakfast foods	Preserves	Salt Pork
Other cereal	Jellies	Bacon
products	Dried fruits	Margarine
Tapioca	Candy	Vegetable and
Sago	Cake and Cookies	nut oils
Potatoes	Other sweet	Peanut Butter
Beans and Peas	desserts	Cheese
Macaroni	Syrup	

Protein Rich Foods	Roughage (regulating foods)
Milk	Raw and Cooked
Eggs	vegetables
Cheese	Cooked cereals
Lean Meat	Cooked and raw fruits
Fish	
Poultry	
Dried Peas	
and Beans	
Legumes	
Nuts	

Protective foods which may be used to build up various body building nutrients are listed below beneath the vitamin they furnish.

PROTECTIVE FOODS HIGH IN VITAMIN CONTENT

Vitamin A	Vitamin B$_1$ (Thiamin)	Vitamin C (Ascorbic Acid)
Codliver oil (tsp)	Pork, lean	Rutabaga (cooked)
Liver	Peanuts	Spinach and
Greens, raw,	Squash	mustard greens
cooked	Whole Wheat	Strawberries
Pumpkin	Nuts	Pimientos (1 tbsp.)
Sweet potato	Wheat germ	Orange juice
Carrots	(1 tbsp.)	Grapefruit juice
Apricots	Apricots and	Cantaloupe
Squash	Peaches	Cauliflower

Green vege-
  tables
Cheese
Pimiento (1 tbsp.)
Tomatoes (raw)
Cream
Corn
Tomato Juice
Egg
Peas, creamed,
  canned
Butter

Asparagus
Dried Beans
Sweet Corn
Turnip tops
Bread-whole
  wheat (enriched)
Liver
Raisins
Oysters
Potatoes (baked)
Milk
Grapefruit
Tomato juice
Oatmeal

Turnips
Peppers, sweet
Asparagus
Other cooked
  greens and green
  vegetables
Tomatoes
Raw green leaves

Iron
Liver
Molasses
Beef heart
Apricots (dried)
Prunes-fresh or
  canned
Nuts
Turkey
Dried fruit
Lean Meat
Eggs
Dried beans
Green leaves
Whole wheat
Oysters
Green vegetables
Dark corn syrup
Peas
Potatoes
Oatmeal

Vitamin B$_2$
(Riboflavin)
Liver
Turnip Tops
Eggplant
Prunes
Sardines
Peanuts
Lean Meats
Dried peaches
Salmon (canned)
Green cooked
  peas
Milk
Beans (dried)
Cantaloupe

Vitamin D
Sea fish oils
Steenbock process
  irradiated foods
Sea foods
To a less degree in
  egg yolk
Butter

Niacin
Liver
Kidney
Heart
Muscle meat
Chicken
Peanuts
Whole wheat
Enriched flour
Beans
Carrots
Oatmeal
Potatoes

A SIMPLE GUIDE FOR MEAL PLANNING

A daily food guide, listing the quantities and kinds of food to use daily to supply body needs, includes:

Milk—1 quart for children, 2 or more cups for adults.

Butter—1 ounce (1 tablespoon); 2 ounces, if skimmed milk is used.

Vegetables—1 serving potatoes, 2 generous servings other vegetables (one raw or leafy).

Fruits—2 servings (one high in vitamin C).

Whole cereals—1 serving: whole grain breakfast cereal, 3-6 slices of bread, muffins, etc., whole grain or enriched.

Meat, poultry, cheese, fish or beans, peas, nuts: 1 or more servings (liver and sea fish once a week).

Eggs— 1 daily (at least 3 to 5 each week).

MENU SUGGESTIONS

ENTREES

Italian Spaghetti
and Meat Balls
Chili Con Carne,
Mexican Style
Braised Beef and
Vegetables
Creamed Ham
and Eggs
Ham Fritters,
Pineapple Sauce
Ham and Macaroni
Au Gratin
Ham and Rice with
Spanish Sauce
Boiled Ham and
Lima Beans
Baked Noodles,
Ham
Escalloped Potatoes
with Ham
Boiled Spareribs,
Red Cabbage
Beef Chop Suey,
Steamed Rice
Potted Sirloin of Beef
Stuffed Green Peppers
Roast Beef Hash
with Potatoes
Corned Beef Hash with

Poached Eggs
Beef Pot Roast
with Noodles
Baked Meat Loaf
Browned Beef Stew
Hungarian Goulash
with Dumplings
Swiss Steak with
Buttered Noodles
Creamed Chipped
Beef with Rice
Creamed Chipped
Beef on Toast
Salisbury Steak with
Browned Onions
Ham and Rice Cakes,
Tomato Sauce
Barbecued Beef on
Bun
Barbecued Pork on
Bun
Broiled Canadian
Bacon
Pork Chop Suey,
Steamed Rice
Creamed Ham and
Green Peppers
Ham Cutlet with
Grilled Tomatoes

Cabbage Rolls
Stuffed with Ham
Veal Fricassee with
Biscuit
Veal Chop Suey,
Steamed Rice
Baked Pork and Bean
Casserole
Chicken Chopped
Salad
Chicken Loaf
Scalloped Chicken
and Macaroni
Lamb Shortcake
with Fresh Peas
Brown Lamb Hash
with Green Peppers
Chopped Beef and
Spaghetti
Turkey Fritters and
Apple Rings
Spaghetti with Mush-
room Sauce
Baked Lima Beans
with Pork
Veal Pot Pie, Flaky
Crust
Irish Lamb Stew,
Dumplings

LAMB

Roast Leg of Lamb,
Mint Jelly
Shepherd Pie
Minced Parsley
Braised Lamb Shank
Boneless Saddle of
Lamb
Baked Lamb Loaf
with Buttered
Noodles
Pan Fried Lamb
Patties
Irish Lamb Stew

Grilled Lamb Chops
Crown Roast of Lamb
Boiled Leg of Lamb,
Horseradish Sauce
Boneless Loin Lamb
Chops
Stuffed Bake Lamb
Chops, Sausage
Stuffing
Breaded Lamb Chops
Pan Fried
Rolled Roast of Lamb,
Rice Stuffing

Lamb and Vegetable
Casserole
Lamb Pot Pie with
Hot Baking Pow-
der Biscuit
Fricassee of Lamb
Stuffed Shoulder of
Lamb, Brown
Sauce
Baked Lamb Loaf,
Tomato Sauce
Lamb Croquettes,
Cream Sauce
Baked Lamb Hash

VEAL

Stuffed Breast of Veal Bread Stuffing
Danish Meat Balls
Chopped Veal Steak
Choice Roast Leg of Veal
Pot Roast of Veal, Vegetables
Crown of Veal Roast

Stuffed Cushion of Veal Brown Sauce
Veal Chops with Buttered Noodles
Pan-Broiled Veal Steak, Mushroom Sauce
Scallopini of Veal
Baked Veal and Ham Loaf, Dill Pickle

Breaded Veal Cutlets, Tomato Sauce
Minced Veal with Green Peppers
Veal Chops with Spanish Sauce
Baked Veal Pie, Hot Biscuits

BEEF

Italian Spaghetti with Meat Balls
Creole Beef with Buttered Noodles
Beef ala Mode with Natural Gravy
Country Fried Steak, Smothered Onions
Baked Salisbury Steak, Spanish Sauce
Boiled Beef with Buttered Noodles
Cold Sliced Beef Plate, Potato Salad
Roast Prime Ribs of Beef, Au Jus
Baked Hamburger Casserole
Baked Hash Vegetable Casserole
Grilled Frankfurters with Spanish Rice
Pan Fried Baby Beef Liver, Bacon
Stuffed Peppers with Tomato Sauce
Creamed Chipped Beef on Toast Points
Yankee Pot Roast with Fresh Vegetables
Boiled Corned Beef and Cabbage
Standing Rib of Beef, Au Jus
Meat Balls and Lima Bean Casserole
Escalloped Hamburger with Potatoes
Braised Flank Steak, Buttered Mushrooms
Home-Made Vegetable Beef Stew

Baked Beef Cutlets, Hungarian Sauce
Choice Top Sirloin Steak, Mushroom Sauce
Braised Round Steak, Swiss Style
Southern Beef Hash with Whipped Yams
American Chop Suey
Beef Pot Pie, Flaky Crust
Hamburger Patties with Boston Baked Beans
Braised Swedish Meat Balls
Baked Corn Beef Hash
Fricassee of Beef, Steamed Rice
Spanish Rice Casserole with Hamburger
Baked Frankfurters with Hot Potato Salad
Simmered Beef Shanks with Parsley Potatoes
Boiled New England Dinner
Baked Swiss Steak, Tomato Sauce
Chili con Carne, Steamed Rice
New England Beef Stew, Boiled Potatoes
Grilled Cubed Steak, Onion Sauce
Baked Shortribs, Barbecue Sauce
Baked Swiss Steak with Dumplings
Beef Kidney Stew, Maryland Style
Baked Beef and Macaroni Loaf, Creole Style
Spanish Meat Loaf
Creamed Chipped Beef on Hot Corn Bread

BEEF (cont.)

Cold Sliced Beef Plate,
  Sliced Tomatoes
Baked Meat Loaf, Brown Gravy
Broiled Sirloin Steak,
  Mushroom Sauce
Boiled Weiners with German
  Sauerkraut

Cold Sliced Beef Tongue
  with Cole Slaw
Porterhouse Steak
Rib Steak
Club Steak
T-Bone Steak

PORK

Roast Loin of Pork
  Baked Apple Rings
Baked Virginia Ham,
  Raisin Sauce
Breaded Pork Tenderloin
Baked Ham Loaf,
  Mustard Sauce
Stuffed Pork Shoulder,
  Applesauce
Broiled Pork Chops,
  Spiced Apple
Grilled Ham Steak,
  Pineapple
Baked Spareribs,
  Barbecue Sauce
Breaded Pork Chops,
  Cream Sauce
Baked Pork Loaf,
  Tomato Sauce
Chipped Ham on Toast
  with Melted Cheese
Ham Croquettes, Cream Sauce
Ham ala King with Hot
  Corn Bread
Baked Ham Souffle with
  Mushrooms
Roast Leg of Pork,
  Applesauce
Boiled Spareribs with
  German Sauerkraut
Boiled Ham and Cabbage
Barbecued Pork Chops
Polish Sausage with
  Sauerkraut
Deviled Pork Chops,
  Glazed Carrots

Jellied Pork Loin,
  Mustard Mayonnaise
Pickled Pig's Feet, Relish
Baked Sugar Cured Ham,
  Cumberland Sauce
Rice and Bacon Casserole,
  Creole Sauce
Breaded Pork Cutlets,
  Glazed Fruit
Cold Pork in Aspic
  Hartford Sauce
Cold Sliced Pork
  Parsley Potatoes
Baked Pork and Bean
  Casserole
Baked Ham with
  Lima Beans
Roast Fresh Pork, Glazed
  Apple Rings
Sliced Cold Boiled Ham
  Sweet Mustard
Smoked Pork Shoulder
Boiled Smoked Pork Jowl,
  Cabbage Wedges
Pork, Cheese and Noodle
  Casserole
Roast Fresh Ham,
  Apple Butter
Baked Pork with Boston
  Baked Beans
Casserole of Pork Steak
  with Riced Potatoes
Scalloped Ham and
  Sweet Potatoes
Cabbage Rolls Stuffed
  with Ham

Diced Ham with Scalloped
    Potatoes
Pork Steak with Country Gravy
Ham Salad on Fruit Plate
Grilled Ham on Toast with
    Cheese Sauce
Fried Pork Liver with
    Grilled Bacon
Ham and Macaroni
Ham Fritters with Pineapple
    Sauce
Creamed Ham and Eggs
Broiled Canadian Bacon
Pork Chop Suey with
    Steamed Rice
Stuffed Pepper with Ham
    and Rice

Cold Baked Ham with
    Potato Salad
Breaded Pork Sausage Patties
Old Fashioned Pork Pie,
    Flaky Crust
Pork Chow Mein, Crispy
    Chinese Noodles
Ham Loaf with Pineapple
    Glaze
Baked Sausages with Whipped
    Potatoes
Ragout of Fresh Pork,
    Hungarian Style
Fluffy Ham Omelette
Noodles with Bacon Strips
Baked Spareribs with
    Buttered Noodles

MEATLESS MAIN DISHES

Macaroni and Eggs with
    Cream Sauce
Baked Macaroni Loaf
Cheese Noodle Loaf
Mexican Spaghetti
Creamed Macaroni with
    Baked Tomatoes
Cabbage Rolls with
    Buttered Noodles
Shrimp Chow Mein
Stuffed Cabbage with Rice
Shrimp and Corn Casserole
Creamed Asparagus on Toast
Home-Baked Beans
Escalloped Cheese and Corn
Corn Fritters
Eggs ala King
Spanish Omelet
Cheese Fondue
Eggs Creamed on Toast
Baked Lima Beans with
    Mushrooms
Chinese Omelet
Baked Macaroni and Cheese
Cheese Souffle
Rice and Tomato Casserole
Vegetable Souffle

Creole Spaghetti
Stuffed Peppers with Rice,
    Tomato Sauce
Escalloped Eggs with Green
    Beans
Rice Croquettes
Eggs, Au Gratin
Welsh Rarebit
Scrambled Eggs
Spanish Rice
Baked Vegetable Pie
Tuna Noodle Casserole
Mushroom Vegetable
    Casserole
Corn Fritters
Potato Pancakes
Mock Chicken Rice with
    Tuna
Vegetable Chop Suey
Baked Lasagna
Creamed Eggs and Shrimp
Macaroni Hash
Egg Cutlets, Cream Sauce
Corn Pudding
Spicy Apple Fritters
Cheese Custard
Cheese Pancakes

MEATLESS MAIN DISHES (cont.)

FISH AND SEAFOOD

New England Codfish Cakes
Baked Fresh Haddock,
  Butter Sauce
Broiled Halibut Steak
Baked Stuffed Mackerel
Poached Salmon Steaks
Pan Fried Perch
Baked Fillets of Fish with
  Spanish Sauce
Creamed Codfish on Toast
Deviled Salmon with Macaroni
Creamed Tuna Fish with Hot
  Buttered Biscuits
Salmon and Potato Casserole
Creamed Salmon with Celery
  and Peas
Tuna Fish ala King
Broiled Maine Lobster
French Fried Oysters
Escalloped Salmon with Eggs
Lobster Newburg
Lobster Thermidor
Baked Salmon Loaf
Tuna Fish and Cheese
  Biscuit Roll

Escalloped Oysters
Baked Scallops in Casserole
Baked Tuna Fish Pie
Seafood Newburg
French Fried Scallops
Shrimp Chop Suey
Tunafish Salad
Salmon Salad
French Fried Shrimp
Baked Salmon Patties
Shrimp Fondue
Tuna Fish Roll
Clam Fricassee
Tuna and Cheese Biscuit Roll
Baked Shrimp and Tuna Newburg
Oyster Pie
Baked Haddock Fillets in
  Spanish Sauce
Broiled Scallops
Fish Sticks with Tartar Sauce
Barbecued Salmon Steaks
Shrimp with Tomato Sauce
Steamed Oysters in the Shell
Tuna Potato Scallop
Fish Stick Burgers

VEGETABLES

Crumbed Cauliflower
Scalloped Green Beans
Boiled Red Cabbage
Stewed Whole Corn
Candied Yams
Glazed Whole Carrots
Fresh Spinach with
  Hard Boiled Egg
Harvard Beets
Buttered Green Asparagus
Baked Succotash
Scalloped Tomatoes with
  Cheese Sauce
Creamed Peas and Carrots
Diced Buttered Turnips
Cold Wax Beans with Vinegar
Mashed Sweet Potatoes on
  Pineapple

Buttered Carrot Strips
Buttered Baby Whole Beets
Boiled Onions with Cheese Sauce
Buttered June Peas
Carrots, Shoestring Style
Corn and Tomato Casserole
Buttered Broccoli with Lemon
  Butter
Spinach
Freshly Cooked Lima Beans
Creamed Cabbage
Creamed Celery
Buttered Corn and Green
  Peppers, Saute
Creamed Small Whole Onions
German Sauerkraut
Stewed Creamed Corn
Baked Corn Pudding

Baked Squash
Stewed Yellow Turnips
Black-Eyed Peas
Baked Stewed Tomatoes
  with Corn
Hot Cole Slaw, Chipped Bacon
Sweet Sour Cabbage
Buttered Brussels Sprouts
Sliced Beets in Orange Sauce
Creamed Broccoli
Baked Stuffed Onions
Corn O'Brien
Baked Shredded Carrots
Corn on the Cob,
  Drawn Butter
Sliced Cucumbers, Vinaigrette
Creamed Mixed Vegetables
Baked Tomatoes Parmesan

Creamed Green Beans
Lima Beans with Tomatoes
Boston Baked Beans
Baked Whole Sweet Potatoes
Braised Carrots
Hot Spiced Beets
Fried Parsnips, Butter Sauce
Au Gratin Carrots
Red Cabbage, German Style
Corn Fritters, Maple Syrup
French Fried Onions
Lyonnaise Carrots
French Fried Eggplant
Baked Beans with Tomatoes
Stewed Navy Beans
Sliced Pickled Beets
Mexican Style Corn with
  Green Peppers

POTATOES

Creamy Whipped Potatoes
Baked Idaho Potato
French Fried Potatoes
Parsley Buttered Potatoes
Hash Brown Potatoes
Hot German Potato Salad
Scalloped Potatoes
Boiled Potatoes
Baked Stuffed Potato
Shoestring Potatoes
Julienne Potatoes
Home Fried Potatoes
Potato Croquettes
German Fried Potatoes
Potato Pancakes
Riced Potatoes

Delmonico Potatoes
Creamed Potatoes
Oven Roasted Potatoes
Potato Dumplings
German Potato Cakes
Chilled Potato Salad,
  Sliced Tomatoes
Potato Chips
Fried Potato Balls
Cottage Fried Potatoes
Potatoes, Au Gratin
Potatoes, O'Brien
Buttered Diced Potatoes
Buttered Steamed Potatoes
Fluffy Mashed Potatoes
Fried Potato Cakes

RICE

Steamed Buttered Rice
Rice Croquettes with
  Mushroom Cream Sauce
Scalloped Rice
Rice Pancakes with
  Maple Syrup

Baked Rice with American
  Cheese
Spanish Rice
Steamed Rice with Tomato
  Sauce
Creamed Rice Casserole

OTHER STARCH FOODS

Boiled Buttered Noodles   Baked Macaroni and Cheese
Macaroni Au Gratin   Macaroni with Tomato Sauce
Chilled Macaroni Salad   Baked Noodles with Spanish Sauce

SUGGESTIONS FOR SALADS

Chilled Fruit Molded Salad
Waldorf Salad
Cole Slaw
Stuffed Celery with Cheese
Cottage Cheese with Sliced
   Tomatoes
Hearts of Lettuce Salad,
   French Dressing
Sliced Cucumber Salad
Grated Carrot and Raisin
   Salad
Pickled Beet and Onion Salad
Chef's Salad
Fruit Salad with Stuffed Prunes
Jellied Vegetable Salad
Egg Salad
Tomato Aspic
Shredded Cabbage and Carrot
   Salad
Perfection Salad
Pineapple Cottage Cheese Salad
Macaroni Salad
Macaroni Coleslaw
Cherry Red Fruit Salad
Jellied Peach Salad
Fruit Salad Ring
Stuffed Beet Salad
Mexican Relish Salad
Wilted Lettuce Salad
Stuffed Pear and Cottage

Cheese Salad
Fresh Fruit Salad,
   Whipped Dressing
Mexican Bean Salad
Carrot Curls with Radish Roses
Shredded Lettuce Salad
Sliced Tomato Salad
Mexican Slaw
Jellied Carrot and Pineapple
   Salad
Deviled Egg Salad
Chilled Macaroni Salad
Head Lettuce with Russian
   Dressing
Chopped Salad Greens,
   Russian Dressing
Stuffed Tomato Salad
Stuffed Prune Salad
Orange and Grapefruit Salad
Asparagus Salad
Sweet-Sour Cucumbers
Mandarin Orange Salad
Jellied Egg Salad
Ginger Ale Fruit Salad
Prune and Cheese Salad
Cabbage, Bacon and Egg
   Salad
String Bean Salad
Frozen Vegetable Salad

SANDWICHES

Lunchmeat Sandwich
Grilled Frankfurter on Bun
Pork Sausage Sandwich
Liverwurst Sandwich
Minced Chicken Sandwich
Sliced Cold Chicken Sandwich
Chicken and Celery Sandwich
Chicken and Ham Sandwich
Chicken Club Sandwich
Egg Salad Sandwich
Hard-Cooked Egg Sandwich
Fried Egg Sandwich
Deviled Egg Sandwich
Scrambled Egg Sandwich
Egg and Celery Sandwich
Egg-Olive-Ham Sandwich
Egg and Bacon Sandwich
Egg and Ham Sandwich
Sardine Sandwich
Tunafish Salad Sandwich
Salmon Salad Sandwich
Shrimp Salad Sandwich
Mock Lobster Salad Sandwich
Fried Oyster Sandwich
Sliced American Cheese
  Sandwich
Toasted Cheese Sandwich
Chopped Cheese and
  Pimiento Sandwich
Grilled Ham Sandwich
Ham and Relish Sandwich
Baked Ham Loaf Sandwich
Minced Ham Sandwich
Ham and Bologna Sandwich
  with Lettuce
Ham and Cheese Sandwich
Ham-Cheese-Pineapple Sandwich
Deviled Ham Sandwich
Cold Roast Beef Sandwich
Cold Sliced Meat Loaf Sandwich

Hot Roast Beef Sandwich
Meat Loaf and Egg Sandwich
Grilled Hamburger on Bun
Grilled Cheeseburger on Bun
Sliced Corned Beef Sandwich
Sliced Cold Lamb Sandwich
Sliced Baked Veal Loaf
  Sandwich
Beef Tongue Sandwich
Mock Chicken Sandwich
Sliced Cold Pork Sandwich
Pickled Beef Tongue Sandwich
Deviled Meat and Prune Sandwich
Bacon, Lettuce and Tomato
  Sandwich
Bologna Sandwich
Cream Cheese Sandwich on
  Brown Bread
Cream Cheese with Sliced Tomato
Cream Cheese and Raisin Nut
  Sandwich
Spiced Veal Sandwich
Shrimp Salad Sandwich with
  Sliced Tomato
Cream Cheese and Egg Salad
  Sandwich
Toasted Peanut Butter Sandwich
Peanut Butter and Jelly Sandwich
Lettuce and Tomato Sandwich
Hot Roast Pork Sandwich
Chicken Salad Sandwich
Cold Meat Salad Sandwich
Barbecued Hamburger on Bun
Hot Hamburger Sandwich with
  Brown Gravy
Sliced Cold Turkey Sandwich
Turkey Salad Sandwich
Barbecued Beef Sandwich
Barbecued Pork Sandwich
Bacon and Cheese Sandwich

QUICK BREAD AND MUFFINS

Baking Powder Biscuits

Buttered Dropped Biscuits

Apple Biscuits

Bacon Biscuits

Buttermilk Biscuits

Sour Milk Biscuits

Hot Bran Biscuits

Butterscotch Biscuits

Lemon Biscuits

Jam and Jelly Biscuits

Honey Biscuits

Cheese Biscuits

Caraway Seed Biscuits

Chopped Fruit Biscuits

Sour Cream Biscuits

Peanut Butter Biscuits

Pineapple Rolls

Hot Orange Biscuits

Hot Cross Buns

Hot Pecan Rolls

Blueberry Muffins

Sour Cherry Muffins

Oven Scones with Raisins

Cherry Nut Bread

Apple Nut Bread

German Coffee Cake

Fruit Bread

Orange-Filled Coffee Cake

Coffee Fruit Ring

Apple Coffee Cake

Apricot Upside-Down
  Coffee Cake

Jam-Filled Breakfast Cake

Old Fashioned Corn Bread

Sour Milk Corn Bread

Pan-Baked Johnny Cake

Hominy Spoon Bread

Corn Sticks

Plain Sugared Doughnuts

Drop Doughnuts

Fruit Doughnuts

Plain Sugar Crullers

Molasses Doughnuts

Rich Dessert Waffles

Hot Griddle Scones

Date and Nut Muffins

Currant Muffins

Cranberry Muffins

Corn Muffins

Brown Sugar Muffins

Bran Nut Muffins

Apricot Muffins

Cinnamon Apple Muffins

Pecan Muffins

Peanut Butter Muffins

Whole Wheat Fruit Muffins

Spiced Prune Muffins

Banana Muffins

Honey Bran Muffins

Molasses Raisin Muffins

Pecan Nut Bread

Date and Nut Bread

Whole Wheat Nut Bread

Orange Date Nut Loaf

Apricot Luncheon Bread

Apricot Bran Bread

Corn Fritters

Blueberry Fritters

Orange Fritters

Apple Fritters

Banana Fritters

Pineapple Fritters

Buttermilk Pancakes

Sour Milk Pancakes

Applesauce Pancakes

Banana Pancakes

Whole Wheat Pancakes

Buckwheat Cakes

Potato Pancakes

Raw Potato Pancakes

Swedish Pancakes

Apple Waffles

Banana Waffles

Nut Waffles

Buttermilk Waffles

Corn Bread Waffles

YEAST BREAD AND ROLLS

Enriched White Bread
Oatmeal Bread
Orange Bread
Raisin Bread
Rye Bread
Whole Wheat Bread
Cinnamon Twist Bread
Raised Biscuits
Butterhorns
Cinnamon Buns
Refrigerator Rolls
Marmalade Rolls
Parker House Rolls
Pecan Rolls
Whole Wheat Rolls
Danish Pastry
Baking Powder Biscuits

Buttermilk Biscuits
Cheese Biscuits
Quick Caramel Biscuits
Scones
Whole Wheat Biscuits
Cornbread
Sally Lunn
Butter Rolls
Raisin-Orange Rolls
Cloverleaf Rolls
Orange Pinwheels
Honey Date Rolls
Oatmeal Yeast Rolls
Onion Buns
Crescent Rolls
Hot Cross Buns
Poppy Seed Rolls

CAKES

Fluffy White Cake
Home-Made Chocolate Cake
Banana Whipped Cream Cake
Sour Milk Devil's Food Cake
Coffee Devil's Food Cake
Chocolate Layer Cake
Spice Cake with Raisins
Applesauce Spice Cake
Gingerbread Cake,
   Marshmallow Topping
Maple Cream Cake
Chocolate Nut Cake
Marble Swirl Cake
Orange Layer Cake
Gold Pound Cake
Angel Food Cake
Custard Angel Food Cake
Lemon Angel Food Cake
Jiffy Sponge Cake

Jelly Roll
Chocolate Cream Roll
Rum Sponge Cake
Orange Chiffon Cake
Peppermint Chip Cake
Coconut Cake
Southern Pecan Cake
Strawberry Short Cake
Boston Cream Pie
Light and Dark Fruit Cake
Peach Upside-Down Cake
Pear Upside-Down Cake
Pineapple Upside-Down Cake
Cottage Cheese Cake
Chocolate Chip Cake
Coconut Fluff Cake
Strawberry Cake
Maraschino Party Cake
Peppermint Angel Food Cake

COOKIES AND CUPCAKES

Vanilla Cupcakes
Chocolate Cupcakes
Fruit and Nut Cakes
Cocoa Cupcakes
Marshmallow Cakes
Lady Fingers
Brown Sugar Drop Cookies
Fruit Drop Cookies
Nut Drop Cookies
Coconut Drop Cookies
Coffee Spice Cookies
Refrigerator Nut Cookies
Chocolate Refrigerator Cookies
Butter Cookies
Lemon Cookies
Raisin-Filled Cookies
Chocolate Brownies
Crisp Sugar Cookies
Vanilla Drop Cookies
Sour Cream Cookies
Butterscotch Cookies
Brandy Cookies
Butter Balls

Chocolate Chip Cookies
Vanilla Pinwheels
Crispy Oatmeal Cookies
Oatmeal Molasses Cookies
Oatmeal Drop Cookies
Date-Filled Oat Squares
Crisp Ginger Cookies
Thick Molasses Cookies
Spice Raisin Cookies
Hermits
Rolled Date Cookies
Filled Cookies
Fig Cookies
Pineapple Drops
Peanut Butter Cookies
Honey Bars
Pumpkin Cookies
Coconut Icebox Cookies
Almond Cookies
Coconut Macaroons
Meringue Kisses
Cornflake Macaroons
Russian Nut Balls

PUDDINGS AND DESSERTS

Apple Betty
Apple Dumplings
Baked Fruit Pudding
Coconut Bread Pudding
Indian Pudding
Peach Crumble Dessert
Pineapple Betty
Almond Torte
Date Delight
Baked Cherry Pudding
Cottage Cheese Pudding
Devil's Food Pudding
Blueberry Puff
Chocolate Pudding
Lemon Cake Top Pudding
Blueberry Cobbler
Fruit Shortcake

Baked Winesap Apple
Apricot Whip
Biscuit Tortoni
Whipped Fruit Gelatin
Jellied Caramel Pudding
Baked Rice Pudding
Peach Cobbler
Chocolate Ice Box Pudding
Tapioca Cream
Cottage Pudding
Blanc Mange
Lemon Cream Rice Pudding
Floating Island Pudding
Graham-Cracker Date
  and Nut Pudding
Raisin Pudding
Peach Tapioca

Butterscotch Blanc Mange
Pineapple Custard Pudding
Apple Sauce Custard
Cherry Cobbler
Cantaloupe
Apple Crumble
Baked Prune Pudding
Strawberry Short Cake
Upside-Down Cherry Pudding
Brown Sugar Custard
Maple Pudding
Peanut Butter Custard
Chocolate Fudge Pudding
Raisin Nut Pudding
Lemon Bisque

Spanish Pudding
Pineapple Marshmallow Fluff
Grapenut Pudding
Baked Alaska
Strawberry Whip
Apple Raisin Torte
Brownie Pudding
Coffee Cream Puffs
Cookie Shortcake
Pineapple-Marshmallow Whip
Fruit Cocktail Tapioca
Marshmallow Fruit Mold
Pineapple Crisp
Spicy Apple Sauce Torte
Apple Cobbler

DESSERT SAUCES

Brown Sugar Syrup
Butterscotch Sauce
Caramel Sauce
Cherry Sauce
Chocolate Sauce
Custard Sauce
Foamy Fruit Sauce
Hard Sauce
Marshmallow Sauce
Orange Sauce
Peppermint-Marshmallow
   Sauce
Vanilla Sauce
Hot Fudge Sauce
Lemon Sauce

Cocoa Dessert Sauce
Pineapple Sauce
Brandy Sauce
Maple Sauce
Tutti-Frutti Sauce
Peach Sauce
Apricot Sauce
Raisin Sauce
Rum Sauce
Strawberry Sauce
Wine Sauce
Honey Sauce
Chocolate Mint Sauce
Lemon Cream Sauce
Nutmeg Sauce

PIES

Frosty Almond
Peppermint
Coconut Butterscotch
Lemon Chiffon
Chocolate Cream
Fresh Rhubarb
Lemon Cheese

Cherry
Blueberry
Peach
Peach Cream
Pecan
Pineapple

PIES (cont.)

Hot Mincemeat	Raspberry Cream
Strawberry Chiffon	Pineapple Cream
Banana Cream	Boston Cream
Nesselrode	Cheese
Dutch Apple	Cranberry Chiffon
Fresh Apple	Sour Cream Raisin
Apricot Cream	Raisin-Pineapple
Banana Chiffon	Fruit Glazed
Butterscotch	Butterscotch Pecan
Coconut Cream	Mocha Chiffon
Coconut Custard	Sweet Potato
Chocolate Chiffon	Egg Nog Chiffon
Apricot Pineapple	Chocolate Peppermint Cream
Light Shoo Fly	Cherry Whipped Cream
Blueberry Chiffon	Pumpkin
Rum Cream	Strawberry Rhubarb
Pineapple Custard	Apple Cream
Lemon Fluff	Black Bottom
Rhubarb	Cherry Almond Cream

FRUIT CUPS

Canned fruit cocktail is ready to serve chilled as it comes from the can. Other canned fruits may also be combined for the beginning course. Garnishes are many and add to the appetite-appeal of the starter for the meal.

Fruit Cup Suggestions

Fruit cocktail, creme de menthe
Orange-grapefruit sections, grenadine
Pineapple chunks, melon balls
Fruit cocktail, unpeeled red apple wedges
Peach slices, grapefruit sections, blueberries
Pear chunks, pineapple tidbits, seedless grapes

Garnishes for Fruit Cups

Small ball of Sherbet	Sugar-frosted edge of cup
Strawberry with green stem left on	Sprig of mint
	Lemon or lime wedge
Few berries	Cranberry Sauce

SEAFOOD COCKTAILS

Shrimp, lobster, crab meat, tuna salmon or a combination may be served chilled and varied in many ways with interesting dressings.

Seafood Cocktail Suggestions
Crabmeat in half avocado
Shrimp and tuna in hollowed-out tomato
Salmon and capers in lettuce-lined sherbet glass
Shrimp and grapefruit sections in watercress nest
Salmon and tart apple wedges
Tuna and quartered deviled egg

Cocktail Dressing Suggestions
Catsup, prepared horseradish
Seafood-chili sauce dressing
Mayonnaise, pickle relish, curry powder
Mayonnaise, chopped chives, tarragon vinegar
Mayonnaise, prepared mustard, prepared horseradish,
      chopped onion and parsley

JUICE COCKTAILS

Both fruit and vegetable juices make excellent first courses when served chilled, just as they come from the can or jar. Garnishes add zest and attractiveness, and may be as simple as mint leaves or a wedge of lime for fruit drinks, or chopped parsley for vegetable ones. They may be more elaborate, such as tiny squares of a frozen whipped cream-horseradish-chopped chives mixture to float on hot consomme and tomato juice.

Fruit Juice Combinations
Pineapple, grapefruit
Orange juice, apricot nectar,
   ginger-ale
Orange-grapefruit, pepper-
   mint flavor
Cranberry, apple, lemon sherbet
Apple, lime, ginger ale
Grape, lemonade
Unsweetened grapefruit juice,
   syrup from canned fruit

Vegetable Juice Combinations
Vegetable juice cocktail,
   chopped chives
Tomato juice, dash Tabasco
   Worcestershire sauce,
   lemon wedges
Clam, tomato, cold or hot
Sauerkraut, tomato
Consomme, tomato or vege-
   table juice cocktail, hot

Juice with Sherbet Floats—Many combinations of fruit juice and syrup from canned fruits may be featured, spiked with a bit of lemon or lime juice, if needed, and dressed up with a small dipper of sherbet.

Juice Over Fruit—Various fruit cups, such as combinations of grapefruit and orange sections with melon balls, are enhanced when a small quantity of either canned juice or syrup made from canned juice is added.

MEAT AND WHAT TO SERVE WITH IT
Beef

Beef Cut	ROAST
Soup or appetizer	Corn chowder, Split pea, Vegetable
Starchy food	Browned potatoes, Mashed potatoes, Boiled potatoes
Other vegetable	Fresh lima beans, Fried eggplant, Asparagus
Bread, rolls, etc.	Parkerhouse rolls, Bread, Soft bun
Accompaniment	Yorkshire pudding, Sage dressing, Pickles
Salad	Lettuce, Apple and celery, Sliced tomato
Dessert	Lemon pie, Ice cream and cake, Peach shortcake

Beef Cut	POT ROAST
Soup or appetizer	Cream of Celery, Tomato, Potato
Starchy food	Boiled noodles, Baked potatoes
Other vegetable	Buttered carrot strips, Buttered green peas, Buttered succotash
Bread, rolls, etc.	Bread, Cheese biscuits, Hot rolls
Accompaniment	Horseradish, Chili sauce, Pickled onions
Salad	Cabbage and apple, Cucumber and onion, Banana
Dessert	Stewed apricots, Baked custard, Butterscotch Pudding

Beef Cut	STEAK
Soup or appetizer	Cream of asparagus, Bean, Chicken
Starchy food	French fried potatoes, Escalloped potatoes, Hashed brown potatoes
Other vegetable	Fried onions, Cauliflower, Baked corn
Bread, rolls, etc.	Pan rolls, Sour milk biscuits, Hot rolls
Accompaniment	Pickled beets, Carrot sticks, Celery
Salad	Combination sliced cucumber, String bean
Dessert	Coconut cream pie, Chocolate pudding, Baked apple

Beef Cut	STEW
Soup or appetizer	Clam chowder, Tomato consomme, Fruit Juice
Starchy food	Rice, Boiled potatoes, Macaroni

Other vegetable	Onions, Carrots, Rutabagas
Bread, rolls, etc.	Corn bread, Whole wheat bread, White bread
Accompaniment	Piccalilli, Radishes, Spiced crab apples
Salad	Fruit, Pimiento, Raw vegetable
Dessert	Layer cake, Rice pudding, Fruit and cookies

Beef Cut	**CORNED BEEF**
Soup or Appetizer	Rice and tomato, Barley, Cream of Spinach
Starchy food	Boiled potatoes, Parsleyed potatoes, Buttered noodles
Other vegetable	Boiled cabbage, Buttered carrots, Turnips
Bread, rolls, etc.	Rye bread, White bread, Hard rolls
Accompaniment	Mustard sauce, Dill pickles, Marmalade
Salad	Celery, Pineapple, Carrot and raisin
Dessert	Fruit gelatin, Banana pudding, Gingerbread

Beef Cut	**HAMBURGER STEAK**
Soup or appetizer	Lima Bean, Potato and carrot, Cream of Corn
Starchy food	Cream potatoes, Fried potatoes, Au gratin potatoes
Other vegetable	Buttered beets, String beans, Summer squash
Bread, rolls, etc.	Hot biscuits, Raisin bread
Accompaniment	Catsup, Green onions, Jam
Salad	Cole slaw, Lettuce and egg, Beet
Dessert	Bread custard, Chocolate pie, Doughnuts

Lamb

Lamb Cut	**ROAST OR LOAF**
Soup or appetizer	Tomato Juice
Starchy food	Mashed sweet potatoes, Parsleyed potatoes, Browned potatoes
Other vegetable	Buttered broccoli, Mashed turnips, Fritter fried egg plant
Bread, rolls, etc.	Parkerhouse rolls, Bread, Soft bun
Accompaniment	Mint sauce, Mint jelly, Assorted pickles
Salad	Macedoine of vegetables, Carrot and pineapple, Lettuce and radish
Dessert	Ice cream and cake, Peach pie, Cornstarch pudding

Lamb Cut	**CHOPS OR PATTIES**
Soup or appetizer	Rice, Beef bouillon, Onion
Starchy food	Lyonnaise potatoes, French fried potatoes, Spanish rice
Other vegetable	New peas, Butter beans, Glazed carrots
Bread, rolls, etc.	Sandwich buns, Raisin bread, Hot rolls

Accompaniment	Tart jelly, Celery-onions, Mint ice
Salad	Bacon-combination, Waldorf, Sliced tomato
Dessert	Berry shortcake, Custard pie, Cantaloupe

Lamb Cut	**STEW**
Soup or appetizer	Puree of green pea, Potato chowder, Fruit cocktail
Starchy food	Steamed rice, Baked noodles, Boiled potatoes
Other vegetable	Julienne green beans, Carrot rings, Buttered lima beans
Bread, rolls, etc.	Hot Biscuits, Corn bread, French bread
Accompaniment	Spiced beets, Radishes, Sour pickles
Salad	Prune and carrot, Vegetable, Pear and grated cheese
Dessert	Bread pudding with chocolate sauce, Berry pie, Apricot tapioca

Veal

Veal Cut	**ROAST**
Soup or appetizer	Puree of bean, Green peas, Consomme
Starchy food	French baked potatoes, Baked sweet potatoes, Mashed potatoes
Other vegetable	Mashed squash, Succotash, Steamed spinach
Bread, rolls, etc.	Bread, Hot rolls, Baking powder biscuits
Accompaniment	Sweet pickles, Raspberry jam, Olives-celery
Salad	Tomato and cucumber, Cabbage and pineapple, Celery and nut
Dessert	Cherry pie, Brown betty, Chocolate ice cream

Veal Cut	**CUTLETS OR CHOPS**
Soup or appetizer	Noodle, Barley and tomato, Vegetable, Lentil, Chicken and rice, Cream of tomato
Starchy food	French baked potatoes, Baked sweet potatoes, Mashed potatoes, Escalloped potatoes
Other vegetable	Harvard beets, Carrots and peas, Wax beans, Carrots and onions, Peas, Braised celery
Bread, rolls, etc.	Bread, Parkerhouse rolls, Finger rolls, Graham Bread
Accompaniment	Cranberry sauce, Tomato sauce, Currant jelly
Salad	Peach and cottage cheese, Lettuce, Asparagus
Dessert	Apple cobbler, White layer cake, Tapioca pudding

Pork

Pork Cut	**ROAST**
Soup or appetizer	Beef broth, Cream of cabbage, French onion
Starchy food	Whipped potatoes, Buttered diced potatoes, Sweet potatoes
Other vegetable	German sauerkraut, Creamed spinach, Broccoli
Bread, rolls, etc.	Bread, Hot rolls, Raisin bread
Accompaniment	Applesauce, Brown gravy, Tart jelly
Salad	Head lettuce, Cole slaw, Banana and nut
Dessert	Lemon ice, Custard pie, Baked pears

Pork Cut	**CHOPS**
Soup or appetizer	Macaroni, Clam juice, Chicken and rice
Starchy food	Cottage fried potatoes, Baked potatoes, French baked potatoes
Other vegetable	Cabbage au gratin, Glazed carrots, Green peas
Bread, rolls, etc.	French bread, Parkerhouse rolls, Graham bread
Accompaniment	Fried apple rings, Marmalade, Celery
Salad	Pineapple and celery, Combination, Sliced tomato
Dessert	Cherry dumplings, Orange gelatin, Spice cake

Pork Cut	**SPARERIBS**
Soup or appetizer	Cream of celery, Tomato, Puree of split pea
Starchy food	Boiled potatoes, French fried sweet potatoes, Mashed potatoes
Other vegetable	Buttered corn on the cob, Buttered mixed vegetables, Buttered wax beans
Bread, rolls, etc.	Corn bread, Hot biscuits, Rye bread
Accompaniment	Apple stuffing, Barbecue sauce, Sliced onions
Salad	Fresh fruit, Cabbage and green pepper, Beet and cucumber
Dessert	Lemon cream pie, Fresh fruit and cookies, Caramel custard

Pork Cut	**BAKED HAM**
Soup or appetizer	Corn chowder
Starchy food	Candied yams, Spanish rice
Other vegetable	Steamed cabbage, Green beans, Asparagus
Bread, rolls, etc.	Vienna bread, Muffins, Bread
Accompaniment	Raisin sauce, Jelly or jam, Radishes, Green onions
Salad	Raw vegetable, Pineapple and cottage cheese
Dessert	Chocolate ice cream, Apricot pie, Fresh fruit and cookies

Pork Cut	**BOILED HAM**
Soup or appetizer	Lentil, Tomato and rice
Starchy food	Mashed sweet potatoes, Parslied potatoes
Other vegetable	Corn pudding, Black-eyed peas, Spinach
Bread, rolls, etc.	Soft bun bread, Pan rolls, Rye bread
Accompaniment	Mustard pickles, Spiced crab apples, Horse-radish
Salad	Apple and date, Onion and cucumber, Cabbage and peanut
Dessert	Banana cream pie, Pineapple ice, Fruit gelatin

Pork Cut	**HAM SLICE**
Soup or appetizer	Pineapple juice, Vegetable, Cream of asparagus
Starchy food	Fried corn meal mush, Baked potatoes, Curried rice
Other vegetable	Baked corn and tomatoes, Fresh lima beans, Creamed carrots
Bread, rolls, etc.	Sour milk biscuits, Bread, Sandwich buns
Accompaniment	Sweet pickles, Cottage cheese, Onion gravy
Salad	Apple, celery and nut, Hearts of lettuce, Tomato
Dessert	Rhubarb pie, Coconut custard, Lemon loaf cake

Pork Cut or Meat Dish	**SAUSAGE**
Soup or appetizer	Puree of potato, Noodle, Macaroni and tomato
Starchy food	Creamed potatoes, Baked sweet potatoes, Fried potatoes
Other vegetable	Hot spiced beets, Boston baked beans, Mexican style corn with green pepper
Bread, rolls, etc.	Corn bread, Bread, Hard rolls
Accompaniment	Browned pineapple, Milk gravy, Watermelon pickles
Salad	Green bean, Carrot and raisin, Spinach and hard-cooked egg
Dessert	Apple pie, Chocolate cake, Chilled melon

MISCELLANEOUS

Meat dish	**CHILI**
Soup or appetizer	Tomato, Cream of potato, Beef broth
Starchy food	Buttered diced potatoes, Steamed rice, Baked potatoes
Other vegetable	Broccoli, Green Beans, Vinegar, Spinach
Bread, Rolls, etc.	French bread, Hard rolls, White bread
Accompaniment	Pickled beets, Dill pickles, Carrot sticks
Salad	Green pepper, Lettuce and tomato, Celery
Dessert	Gelatin and oatmeal cookies, Coconut layer cake

Meat dish	**FRANKFURTERS**
Soup or appetizer	Oyster stew, Split pea, Cream of corn
Starchy food	Hot potato salad, Spanish rice, Baked Macaroni
Other vegetable	Steamed sauerkraut, Baked beans, Whole kernel corn
Bread, rolls, etc.	Rye bread, Sandwich buns, Bread
Accompaniment	Barbecue sauce, Mustard, Catsup
Salad	Cabbage and pineapple, Beet and onion, Sliced tomato
Dessert	Apricot brown betty, Pineapple tapioca, Strawberry shortcake

Meat dish	**MEAT LOAF**
Soup or appetizer	Consomme, Puree of white bean, Tomato juice
Starchy food	Lyonnaise potatoes, Hashed in cream potatoes, Curried rice
Other vegetable	Black-eyed peas, Fried eggplant, Creamed onions
Bread, rolls, etc.	Finger rolls, Graham bread, Corn bread
Accompaniment	Spanish sauce, Chili sauce, Mustard pickles
Salad	Fruit, Combination, Carrot, prune and celery
Dessert	Jelly roll, Coffee ice cream, Peach cobbler

Meat dish	**HEART**
Soup or appetizer	Navy bean, Vegetable chowder, Onion
Starchy food	Buttered noodles, Candied yams, Fried potatoes
Other vegetable	Boiled onions, Fried corn, Escalloped tomatoes
Bread, rolls, etc.	Parkerhouse rolls, Baking powder biscuits, Bread
Accompaniment	Sage stuffing, Spiced gooseberries, Currant jelly
Salad	Cole slaw, Asparagus, Combination Fruit
Dessert	Apricots and brownies, Prune whip, Raisin pie

Meat dish	**LIVER**
Soup or appetizer	Tomato juice, Spring vegetable, Celery
Starchy food	French fried potatoes, Potatoes in jackets, Steamed brown rice
Other vegetable	Hot slaw, Lima beans, French fried onions
Bread, rolls, etc.	White bread, Raisin bread, Hot rolls
Accompaniment	Bacon, Pickled onions, Assorted pickles
Salad	Pineapple and cheese, Endive, Banana
Dessert	Pumpkin pie, Peaches and cream, Cup cakes

Meat dish	**TONGUE**
Soup or appetizer	Noodle, Beef broth with rice
Starchy food	Boiled potatoes, Mashed potatoes, Escalloped potatoes
Other vegetable	Steamed spinach, Wax beans, Braised celery
Bread, rolls, etc.	Rye bread, Hard rolls, Bread
Accompaniment	Raisin sauce, Spanish sauce, Horseradish
Salad	Spiced beet, Pineapple, Lettuce
Dessert	Chocolate pudding, Mince pie, Ice cream with fruit sauce

Meat dish	**ASSORTED COLD MEATS**
Soup or appetizer	Clam chowder, Bean puree, Onion au gratin
Starchy food	Potato salad, Macaroni, Creamed whole potatoes
Other vegetable	Sliced jumbo tomatoes, Sliced cucumbers vinaigrette, Succotash
Bread, rolls, etc.	Cheese biscuits, Bread, Parkerhouse rolls
Accompaniment	Sweet pickles, Sliced cheese, Mustard pickles
Salad	Shredded lettuce, Fruit, String bean and celery
Dessert	Apple turnovers, Rhubarb sauce and cookies, Cottage pudding

Menus for 52 Weeks

1st Week

SUNDAY

BREAKFAST
Chilled Melon
Scrambled Eggs
Hickory Smoked
  Bacon
Cinnamon Raisin
  Pecan Rolls
Beverage(s)

DINNER
Cranberry Juice
Fried Chicken
Mashed Potatoes
Buttered Asparagus
Jellied Pineapple and
  Carrot Salad
Clover Leaf
  Rolls
Butter of Margarine
Sponge Cake
  with Vanilla Sauce
Beverage(s)

SUPPER
Celery Soup
Assorted Cold Cuts
Tomato Slice
Cole Slaw
Potato Chips
Bread
Butter or Margarine
Catsup-Mustard
Old Fashioned
  Molasses
   Cookies
Beverage(s)

MONDAY

BREAKFAST
Assorted Fruit Juices
Selected Cold Cereals
  or
Oatmeal with Cream
Toast, Buttered
Jelly
Beverage(s)

DINNER
Cherry Juice
Salisbury Steak
Browned Potatoes
Buttered Green Beans
Mixed Vegetable Salad

Bread, white and dark
Butter or Margarine
Fruit Gelatin Dessert
Beverage(s)

SUPPER
Split Pea Soup
Grilled Ham Sand-
  wich
Pickles
Carrot and Raisin
  Salad
Spice Cake
Beverage(s)

TUESDAY

BREAKFAST
  Orange Sections
  Poached Egg on
    Buttered Toast
  Hot Rolls
  Butter or Margarine
  Jam
  Beverage(s)

DINNER
  Apple Juice
  Pork Roast
  Glazed Sweet
    Potatoes
  Tomatoes with
    Celery Sauce
  Perfection
    Salad
  Cornbread
  Butter or Margarine
    and Jam
  Baked Custard
  Beverage(s)

SUPPER
  Spanish Rice with
    Chopped Meat
  Fruit Slaw
  Bread, white and dark
  Butter or Margarine
  Lemon Oatmeal
    Drop Cookies
  Beverage(s)

WEDNESDAY

BREAKFAST
  Bananas with Cream
  Golden French Toast
  Maple Syrup or Honey
  Canadian Bacon
  Beverage(s)

DINNER
  Chicken Pie
  Broccoli, buttered
  Spiced Peaches
  Bread, white and dark
  Butter or Margarine
  Chocolate Pudding
  Beverage(s)

SUPPER
  Beef Rice Soup
  Egg Salad Sandwiches
    (white and dark
    bread)
  Apple and Cheese
    Wedges
  Prune Whip
  Beverage(s)

THURSDAY	FRIDAY

BREAKFAST
Assorted Juices
Selected Cold Cereal
or
Wheatena with Cream
Corn Muffins
Butter or Margarine
Jelly
Beverage(s)

DINNER
Baked Ham
Carrot Slices
Boiled Potatoes
Jellied Perfection
Salad
Bread, white and dark
Butter or Margarine
Butterscotch Ice-
Box Cookies
Beverage(s)

SUPPER
Vegetable Soup
Fricassee of Lamb
on Hot Biscuit
Tossed Green Salad
with Italian
Dressing
Chilled Pear Halves
Beverage(s)

BREAKFAST
Grapefruit Half
Fried Eggs
Plantation Sausage
Toast
Butter or Margarine
Jam
Beverage(s)

DINNER
Fried Scallops with
Tartar Sauce
Parslied Buttered
Potatoes
Green Beans
Sunshine Salad
Bread, white and dark
Butter or Margarine
Lemon Meringue Pie
Beverage(s)

SUPPER
Cream of Vichoyoisse
Soup
Tomato Stuffed with
Tuna Salad
Potato Chips
Hot Rolls
Butter or Margarine
Pineapple Chunks
Chilled
Beverage(s)

SATURDAY

BREAKFAST
Assorted Juices
Buttermilk Pancakes
Honey Butter
Warm Maple Syrup
Grilled Ham
Beverage(s)

DINNER
Swiss Steak
Boiled Potatoes
Buttered Cauliflower
Pineapple Slaw
Bread, white and dark
Butter or Margarine
Chilled Peaches
Beverage(s)

SUPPER
French Onion Soup
Toasted Cheese
    Sandwiches with Bacon
Waldorf Salad
Peanut Butter
    Cookies
Beverage(s)

2nd Week

SUNDAY	MONDAY

BREAKFAST
Chilled Orange Juice
Country Fresh Eggs
Grilled Sausages
Almond Nut
   Doughnuts
Butter or Margarine
Beverage(s)

BREAKFAST
Fruit in Season
Old Fashioned Waffles
Honey or Maple Syrup
Soft Butter
Beverage(s)

DINNER
Apple Juice
Roast Chicken
Herb Dressing

Mashed Potatoes
Baked Hubbard
   Squash
Jellied Cranberry
   Salad
Clover Leaf Rolls
Butter or Margarine
Raspberry Sherbet—
   Cookies
Beverage(s)

DINNER
Roast Veal
Browned Potatoes
Barbecued Lima Beans
Pineapple and Carrot
   Salad
Rolls
Butter or Margarine
Chocolate Cake
Beverage(s)

SUPPER
Tomato-Rice
   Bouillon
Ham and Cheese
   Sandwiches, (dark
   and white bread)
Relish Tray
Apple Crisp
Beverage(s)

SUPPER
Split Pea Soup
Turkey Salad
Tomato Slices
Bread, white and dark
Butter or Margarine—
   Jelly
Vanilla Pudding—
   Caramel Sauce
Beverage(s)

TUESDAY	**WEDNESDAY**

BREAKFAST
   Assorted Juices
   Poached Egg on
     Buttered Toast
   Orange Pineapple
     Danish Roll
   Butter or Margarine
   Jelly
   Beverage(s)

BREAKFAST
   Grapefruit Half
   Selected Cold Cereal
     or
   Cream of Wheat,
     with Cream
   Golden Toast
   Butter or Margarine
   Jelly
   Beverage(s)

DINNER
   Salisbury Steak
   Scalloped Potatoes

   Asparagus
   Chopped Cole
     Slaw
   Bread, white and dark
   Butter or Margarine
   Chilled Pears
   Beverage(s)

DINNER
   Roast Beef and Gravy
   Mashed Potatoes
   Broccoli, buttered
   Beet Salad
   Muffins
   Butter or Margarine
   Applesauce Cake
   Beverage(s)

SUPPER
   Consomme
   French Toast
   Escalloped Apples
   Pork Sausage Links

   Ice Cream—Cookies
   Beverage(s)

SUPPER
   Creamed Celery Soup

   Broiled Hamburger Sand-
     wich
   Cole Slaw
   Potato Chips
   Catsup-Mustard-Onions
   Butterscotch Ice Box
     Cookies
   Beverage(s)

THURSDAY

BREAKFAST
Chilled Fruit Juice
Buttermilk Pancakes
Soft Butter
Warm Maple Syrup
  or Honey
Beverage(s)

DINNER
Meat Loaf
Potatoes au Gratin

Green Beans
Rolls
Butter or Margarine
Fresh Orange Cake
Beverage(s)

SUPPER
Vegetable Soup

Cheese Rarebit with
  Bacon on Toast
Lettuce Salad/
  dressing
Peach Tapioca
  Pudding
Beverage(s)

FRIDAY

BREAKFAST
Orange Slices
Scrambled Eggs
Crisp Bacon
Toast
Butter or Margarine
Jelly
Beverage(s)

DINNER
Tomato Juice
Oven Fried Ocean
  Perch Fillets
Scalloped Potatoes

Brussel Sprouts,
  buttered
Shredded Lettuce
  Salad/dressing

Brownies
Beverage(s)

SUPPER
Clam Chowder
Savory Shrimp and
  Rice Casserole
Cabbage and Green
  Pepper Salad
Rolls
Butter or Margarine
Chilled Pineapple
  Chunks
Beverage(s)

SATURDAY

BREAKFAST
   Stewed Prunes,
     Lemon Slices
   Assorted Cold Cereals
       or
   Oatmeal with Cream
   Cinnamon Streusel
     Danish
   Butter or Margarine
   Beverage(s)

DINNER
   Hungarian Goulash
     with Noodles
   Royal Orange and
     Apple Salad
   French Bread
   Butter or Margarine
   Coconut Custard Pie

   Beverage(s)

SUPPER
   Individual Chicken Pies

   Head Lettuce with
     Fruits
   Cloverleaf Rolls
   Butter or Margarine
   Chocolate Pudding,
     Whipped Cream
   Beverage(s)

3rd Week

SUNDAY	MONDAY
BREAKFAST	**BREAKFAST**
Grapefruit and Orange Sections	Chilled Fruit Juice
Bacon Omelet	Assorted Cold Cereals
Golden Toast	or
Butter or Margarine	Wheatena, with Cream
Jam or Marmalade	Cheese Danish Roll
Beverage(s)	Butter or Margarine
	Beverage(s)

BREAKFAST
Grapefruit and
  Orange Sections
Bacon Omelet
Golden Toast
Butter or Margarine
Jam or Marmalade
Beverage(s)

DINNER
Veal Roast
Fluffy Mashed
  Potatoes
Cauliflower a la
  Creole
Cucumber and Onion
  Salad
Rolls
Butter or Margarine
Apple Pie a la
  Mode
Beverage(s)

SUPPER
Chicken Noodle
  Soup
Assorted Sandwiches
  (Egg, Cheese,
  Ham, Chicken)
Raw Vegetable Tray
Chocolate Eclair
Beverage(s)

BREAKFAST
Chilled Fruit Juice
Assorted Cold Cereals
  or
Wheatena, with Cream
Cheese Danish Roll
Butter or Margarine
Beverage(s)

DINNER
Baked Ham
Baked Squash
Creamed Spinach
Bread, white and dark
Butter or Margarine
Cabbage and Green
  Pepper Salad
Orange Cake
Beverage(s)

SUPPER
Beef Vegetable Soup
Chicken Chow Mein
Fluffy White Rice
Cottage Cheese and
  Pineapple Salad
Apple Strudel
Beverage(s)

TUESDAY

BREAKFAST
  Stewed Apricots
  Fried Egg
  Hickory Smoked
    Bacon
  Golden Toast
  Butter or Margarine
  Jam
  Beverage(s)

DINNER
  Swiss Steak
  Parsley Buttered
    Potatoes
  Harvard Beets
  Corn Relish
  Bread, white and
    dark
  Butter or Margarine
  Steamed Prune
    Pudding
  Beverage(s)

SUPPER
  Ham Chowder
  Deviled Egg and
    Olive Sandwich
    Filling
    (dark and light
    bread)
  Scalloped
    Tomatoes
  Jellied Pineapple
    and Carrot Salad
  Banana Cake
  Beverage(s)

WEDNESDAY

BREAKFAST
  Chilled Pineapple Juice
  Assorted Cold Cereals
    or
  Oatmeal with Cream
  Hot Rolls
  Butter or Margarine
  Jelly
  Beverage(s)

DINNER
  Beef Pot Roast and
    Gravy
  Browned Potatoes
  Lima Beans in Butter
    Sauce
  Green Salad/dressing

  Bread, white and
    dark
  Butter or Margarine
  Snow Pudding
  Beverage(s)

SUPPER
  Apple Juice
  French Toast
  Hot Syrup
  Sausage Patties
  Chilled Pineapple
    Chunks—Cookies
  Beverage(s)

THURSDAY	FRIDAY

BREAKFAST
Grapefruit Sections
  Grenadine
Poached Egg on
  Buttered Toast
Apple Danish Roll
Butter or Margarine
Beverage(s)

BREAKFAST
Chilled Prune Juice
Old Fashioned Waffles
Honey Butter
Warm Maple Syrup
Beverage(s)

DINNER
Yankee Pot Roast
Fresh Vegetables
Apple Nut Salad

Bread, dark and white
Butter or Margarine
Iced Yellow Cup
  Cakes
Beverage(s)

DINNER
Fried Ocean Perch
  Fillets
Baked Rice
Asparagus
Sunshine Salad
Bread, white and dark
Butter or Margarine
Grape-Nut Custard
Beverage(s)

SUPPER
Scotch Broth
Macaroni au
  Gratin
Tomato on Shredded
  Lettuce with
  dressing
Warm Rolls
Butter or Margarine
Vanilla Cream
  Pudding,
  Chocolate Sauce
Beverage(s)

SUPPER
Clam Chowder
New England Lasagne
  with Tomato Sauce
Jellied Pineapple and
  Carrot Salad
Rolls
Butter or Margarine
Dutch Apple Pie
Beverage(s)

SATURDAY

BREAKFAST
   Chilled Fresh Melon
     Slice
   Assorted Cold Cereals
       or
   Cream of Wheat,
     warm milk
   Cinnamon Raisin
     Pecan Roll
   Butter or Margarine
   Beverage(s)

DINNER
   Veal Cutlet,
     Mushroom Sauce
   Delmonico Potatoes

   Buttered Green Beans
   Green Salad/dressing

   Pound Cake
   Beverage(s)

SUPPER
   Potato Chowder
   Creamed Chipped Beef
     on Toast
   Crisp Vegetable Salad/
     dressing
   Bread, white and dark
   Butter or Margarine
   Fruited Oatmeal Drops

   Whipped Cherry Gelatin

   Beverage(s)

4th Week

SUNDAY	MONDAY
BREAKFAST	**BREAKFAST**
Chilled Melon	Assorted Fruit Juices
Scrambled Eggs	Selected Cold Cereals
Hickory Smoked	or
Bacon	Oatmeal, with Cream
Cinnamon Raisin	Toast, Buttered
Pecan Rolls	Jelly
Beverage(s)	Beverage(s)
DINNER	**DINNER**
Roast Pork	Meat Loaf
Parsley Buttered	Mashed Potatoes
Potatoes	Buttered Carrot Rings
Chopped Spinach	Pears and Lime Gelatin
with Bacon	Salad
Dressing	Graham Muffins
Apple Sauce	Butter or Margarine
Corn Bread	Peach Tapioca
Butter or Margarine	Beverage(s)
Vanilla Ice Cream—	
Cookies	
Beverage(s)	
SUPPER	**SUPPER**
Tomato-Barley Soup	Split Pea Soup
Assorted Cold Cuts	Creamed Chicken
and Cheese	Almondine
Potato Chips	Hot Biscuits
Relishes	Cabbage, Apple, Raisin
Bread, white and dark	Salad
Butter or Margarine	Lemon Refrigerator
Honey Pecan Tarts	Dessert
Beverage(s)	Beverage(s)

TUESDAY	WEDNESDAY

BREAKFAST
Orange Sections
Poached Egg on
    Buttered Toast
Hot Rolls
Butter or Margarine
Jam
Beverage(s)

BREAKFAST
Bananas with Cream
Golden French Toast
Maple Syrup or Honey
Canadian Bacon
Beverage(s)

DINNER
Baked Ham with
    Raisin Sauce
Glazed Sweet
    Potatoes
Succotash
Clover-Leaf Rolls

Butter or Margarine
Orange Layer Cake
    with Orange
    Butter Icing
Beverage(s)

DINNER
Braised Chicken Legs
    in Sauce
Stuffed Baked Potatoes

Lima Beans
Tossed Green Salad/
    dressing
Bread, white and dark
Butter or Margarine
Peach Chiffon Pudding
Beverage(s)

SUPPER
Vegetable Soup

Ham Salad Sand-
    wich, (white and
    dark bread)
Jellied Tomato Salad

Celery and Carrot
    Sticks
Apple Crisp
Beverage(s)

SUPPER
Tomato Soup
Macaroni and Cheese
Pickled Beet Salad
Cubed Gelatin
Honey-Nut Spice Cake
Beverage(s)

THURSDAY	FRIDAY

BREAKFAST
Assorted Juices
Selected Cold Cereal
    or
Wheatena, with cream
Corn Muffins
Butter or Margarine
Jelly
Beverage(s)

BREAKFAST
Grapefruit Half
Fried Eggs
Plantation Sausage
Toast
Butter or Margarine
Jam
Beverage(s)

DINNER
Baked Spare Ribs
    and Sauerkraut
Boiled Potatoes
Candied Carrot Coins
Cider Fruit Salad
Rolls
Butter or Margarine
Pound Cake-Chilled
    Apple Sauce
Beverage(s)

DINNER
Tuna a la King in
    Pastry Shell
Buttered Peas
Sliced Tomato and
    Lettuce Salad
Rolls
Butter or Margarine
Orange Cup Cakes
Beverage(s)

SUPPER
Puree of Lima Bean
    Soup
Hamburgers on Bun
Relishes
Sliced Tomatoes
    on Lettuce
Custard Pie
Beverage(s)

SUPPER
Manhattan Clam
    Chowder
Welsh Rarebit on
    Buttered Toast

Tossed Green Salad

Blue Plums—Cookies
Beverage(s)

SATURDAY

BREAKFAST
    Assorted Juices
    Buttermilk Pancakes
    Honey Butter
    Warm Maple Syrup
    Grilled Ham
    Beverage(s)

DINNER
    Pan Fried Lamb Patties
    Mashed Potatoes
    Scalloped Corn
    Jellied Vegetable
       Salad
    Rolls
    Butter or Margarine
    Pineapple Chunks
    Beverage(s)

SUPPER
    Minestrone Soup
    Beef and Whipped
       Potato au Gratin
    Waldorf Salad
    Fruit Gelatin with
       Whipped Cream
    Beverage(s)

5th Week

SUNDAY	MONDAY

BREAKFAST
    Chilled Orange Juice
    Country Fresh Eggs
    Grilled Sausages
    Almond Nut
      Doughnuts
    Butter or Margarine
    Beverage(s)

BREAKFAST
    Fruit in Season
    Old Fashioned Waffles
    Crisp Bacon
    Honey or Maple Syrup
    Soft Butter
    Beverage(s)

DINNER
    Cranberry Juice
    Roast Beef and Gravy
    Browned Potatoes
    Lyonnaise Green
      Beans
    Lettuce Wedge
      with dressing
    Rolls
    Butter or Margarine
    Fudge Pudding with
      Topping
    Beverage(s)

DINNER
    New England Boiled
      Dinner   (Corned
      Beef, Cabbage, Boiled
      Parsley Potatoes)
    Bread, white and dark
    Butter or Margarine
    Baked Rice Custard
    Beverage(s)

SUPPER
    Vegetable-Rice Soup
    Chicken Salad
    Sliced Tomatoes
    Stuffed Celery
      Sticks
    Parker House
      Rolls
    Butter or Margarine
    Vanilla Ice Cream—
      Cookies
    Beverage(s)

SUPPER
    Creole Soup
    Assorted Sandwiches
      (Egg, Ham, Cheese,
      Turkey)
    Relishes
    Butterscotch
      Brownies
    Beverage(s)

TUESDAY	WEDNESDAY

BREAKFAST
  Assorted Juices
  Poached Egg on
    Buttered Toast
  Orange Pineapple
    Danish Roll
  Butter or Margarine
  Jelly
  Beverage(s)

DINNER
  Braised Short Ribs—
    Vegetable
  Gravy
  Boiled Potatoes
  Spinach Souffle
  Royal Orange and
    Apple Salad
  Cinnamon Spice Cake
  Beverage(s)

SUPPER
  Ham and Split Pea
    Soup
  Meat Patties
  Hashed Brown
    Potatoes
  Cucumber and
    Onion Salad
  Rolls
  Butter or Margarine
  Chilled Pears—
    Cookies

BREAKFAST
  Half Grapefruit
  Selected Cold Cereal
    or
  Cream of Wheat,
    with cream
  Golden Toast
  Butter or Margarine
  Jelly
  Beverage(s)

DINNER
  Breaded Veal Cutlets
    in Tomatoes
  Scalloped Potatoes

  Harvard Beets
  Pineapple Slaw
    Salad
  Bread, white and dark
  Butter or Margarine
  Apple Cobbler
  Beverage(s)

SUPPER
  Cream of Celery
    Soup
  Beef Pot Pie
  Buttered Carrots
  Rolls, home-made
  Butter or Margarine
  Chocolate Cake
  Beverage(s)

THURSDAY	FRIDAY

BREAKFAST
Chilled Fruit Juice
Buttermilk Pancakes
Soft Butter
Warm Maple Syrup
  or Honey
Beverage(s)

BREAKFAST
Orange Slices
Scrambled Eggs
Crisp Bacon
Toast
Butter or Margarine
Jelly
Beverage(s)

DINNER
Baked Liver covered
  with Bacon
  Strips
Buttered Mashed
  Turnips
Spinach with Chopped
  Bacon Dressing
Oatmeal Rolls
Butter or Margarine
Tomato Aspic with
  Cottage Cheese
Crumb Spice Cake
Beverage(s)

DINNER
Fried Scallops
Potato Puff (Duchess)

Carrot and Raisin Slaw
Crispy Corn Bread
Butter or Margarine
Cherry Gelatin Squares
Beverage(s)

SUPPER
Corned Beef Hash
Buttered Green Beans
Bread, white and dark
Butter or Margarine
Vanilla Pudding with
  Caramel Sauce
Beverage(s)

SUPPER
French Onion
  Soup
Stuffed Peppers in
  Tomato Sauce
Fruit Salad
Buttered Asparagus
Bread
Butter or Margarine
Peaches and Cookies
Beverage(s)

SATURDAY

BREAKFAST
    Stewed Prunes,
       Lemon Slices
    Assorted Cold Cereals
           or
    Oatmeal, with Cream
    Cinnamon Streusel
       Danish
    Butter or Margarine
    Beverage(s)

DINNER
    Lamb Roast with
       Mint Jelly
    Stuffed Baked
       Potatoes
    Buttered Cauliflower
    Perfection Salad
    Bread
    Butter or Margarine
    Butterscotch Bars
    Beverage(s)

SUPPER
    Chicken Rice Soup
    Tuna a la King
    Buttered Corn
    Sunshine Salad
    Cherry Pie
    Beverage(s)

6th Week

SUNDAY	MONDAY

BREAKFAST
Grapefruit and
  Orange Sections
Bacon Omelet
Golden Toast
Butter or Margarine
Jam or Marmalade
Beverage(s)

BREAKFAST
Chilled Fruit Juice
Assorted Cold Cereals
  or
Wheatena, with Cream
Cheese Danish Roll
Butter or Margarine
Beverage(s)

DINNER
Oven Baked
  Chicken Legs
Potatoes au
  Gratin
Buttered Broccoli
Endive Salad/dressing
Rolls, whole wheat or
  graham
Butter or Margarine
Mocha Nut Cake
  with Topping
Beverage(s)

DINNER
Swiss Steak
  Smothered in
  Tomatoes and
  Onions
Browned Potatoes
Buttered Cauliflower
Shredded Lettuce
  Salad/dressing
Roll
Butter or Margarine
Baked Apples
Beverage(s)

SUPPER
English Beef Broth

Cold Meat Cuts
  and Cheese
Relishes, Green and
  Black Olives
Bread, white and dark
Butter or Margarine
Strawberry Ice Cream
Beverage(s)

SUPPER
Ground Beef
  and Spaghetti
Lyonnaise Green Beans
French Bread
Butter or Margarine
Chilled Pears
Beverage(s)

TUESDAY	WEDNESDAY

BREAKFAST
Stewed Apricots
Fried Egg
Hickory Smoked
  Bacon
Golden Toast
Butter or Margarine
Jam
Beverage(s)

DINNER
Liver Creole
Mashed Potatoes
Harvard Beets
Bread, white and dark
Butter or Margarine
Strawberry-Banana
  Mold
Beverage(s)

SUPPER
Vegetable Soup
Toasted Cheese Sandwich
Head Lettuce Salad/
  dressing
Bread, white and dark
Butter or Margarine
Peaches—Cookies
Beverage(s)

BREAKFAST
Chilled Pineapple Juice
Assorted Cold Cereals
  or
Oatmeal, with Cream
Hot Rolls
Butter or Margarine
Jelly
Beverage(s)

DINNER
Ham Patties on a
  Pineapple Slice
Buttered Peas
Hashed Brown Potatoes

Cabbage-Raisin-Nut
  Salad
Bread, white and dark
Butter or Margarine
Cherry Brown Betty

Beverage(s)

SUPPER
Fiesta Hamburgers
Potato Chips
Green Beans
Grapefruit Salad,
  Cherry Topped
Fudge Pudding
Beverage(s)

THURSDAY	FRIDAY
BREAKFAST	**BREAKFAST**
Grapefruit Sections, Grenadine	Chilled Prune Juice
Poached Egg on Buttered Toast	Old Fashioned Waffles
Apple Danish Roll	Honey Butter
Butter or Margarine	Warm Maple Syrup
Beverage(s)	Beverage(s)

DINNER

DINNER	**DINNER**
Apple Juice	V-8 Juice
Roast Chicken and Gravy	Fried Scallops
Buttered Rice	Buttered Spinach
Scalloped Corn	Salad Greens/dressing
Peppy Beet Salad	Plain Muffins
Rolls	Fruit Pudding, served with Hot Custard Sauce
Butter or Margarine	Beverage(s)
Mincemeat Squares	
Beverage(s)	

SUPPER	**SUPPER**
Rice-Tomato Bouillon	Cream of Asparagus Soup
Ham and Egg Salad Plate	Cheese Souffle
Corn Muffins	Lima Beans
Butter or Margarine	Bread, white and dark
Butterscotch Pudding	Butter or Margarine
Beverage(s)	Baked Apples
	Beverage(s)

SATURDAY

BREAKFAST
    Chilled Fresh
        Melon Slice
    Assorted Cold Cereals
            or
    Cream of Wheat,
        warm milk
    Cinnamon Raisin
        Pecan Roll
    Butter or Margarine
    Beverage(s)

DINNER
    Shepherd's Pie
    Buttered Carrots
    Cabbage Relish
    Bread, white and dark
    Butter or Margarine
    Fruit Cup
    Beverage(s)

SUPPER
    Chicken Rice Soup
    Beef Barbecue on Bun
    Potato Salad
    Green Beans
    Chilled Peaches
    Bran Applesauce
        Cookies
    Beverage(s)

7th Week

SUNDAY	MONDAY

BREAKFAST
  Chilled Melon
  Scrambled Eggs
  Hickory Smoked
    Bacon
  Cinnamon Raisin
    Pecan Rolls
  Beverage(s)

DINNER
  Roast Pork Loin
  Mashed Potatoes
  Buttered Green Beans
  Gingerale Fruit Salad

  Homemade Rolls
  Butter or Margarine
  Golden Chiffon Cake/
    Topping
  Beverage(s)

SUPPER
  Tomato Rice
    Bouillon
  Tuna Salad
  Shoestring Potatoes
  Bread, white and dark
  Butter or Margarine
  Easy Mix Cookies
  Beverage(s)

BREAKFAST
  Assorted Fruit Juices
  Selected Cold Cereals
    or
  Oatmeal, with Cream
  Toast, Buttered
  Jelly
  Beverage(s)

DINNER
  Oven Fried Chicken
  Mashed Potatoes
  Baby Lima Beans
  Cabbage and Green
    Pepper Salad
  Rolls
  Butter or Margarine
  Bread Pudding, Fruit
    Sauce
  Beverage(s)

SUPPER
  Vegetable Soup
  Cheese Sandwiches and
    Ham Sandwiches
  Orange, Apple and
    Banana Salad
  Honey-Nut Spice
    Cake
  Beverage(s)

TUESDAY	WEDNESDAY

BREAKFAST
  Orange Sections
  Poached Egg on
    Buttered Toast
  Hot Rolls
  Butter or Margarine
  Jam
  Beverage(s)

BREAKFAST
  Bananas with Cream
  Golden French Toast
  Maple Syrup or Honey
  Canadian Bacon
  Beverage(s)

DINNER
  Baked Lamb Loaf
  Buttered Peas
  Jellied Pineapple
    and Carrot Salad
  Rolls
  Butter or Margarine
  Orange and Raisin
    Cup Cakes
  Beverage(s)

DINNER
  Pot Roast of Beef
  Browned Potatoes
  Buttered Green Peas
  Pear and Cheese
    Salad/dressing
  Butter or Margarine
  Rolls
  Fruited Tapioca
  Beverage(s)

SUPPER
  Chicken Soup
  Bacon, Lettuce and
    Tomato Sandwich
  Potato Chips
  Tossed Salad/dressing

  Butterscotch Pudding—
    Topping
  Beverage(s)

SUPPER
  Cream of Asparagus
    Soup
  Denver Egg Sandwich
  Grated Carrot and
    Peanut Salad
  Chocolate Pudding
  Beverage(s)

THURSDAY	FRIDAY

BREAKFAST
Assorted Juices
Selected Cold Cereal
or
Wheatena, with Cream
Corn Muffins
Butter or Margarine
Jelly
Beverage(s)

BREAKFAST
Grapefruit Half
Fried Eggs
Plantation Sausage
Toast
Butter or Margarine
Jam
Beverage(s)

DINNER
Meat Loaf
Scalloped Potatoes

Shredded Cabbage
Salad
Harvard Beets
Cherry Cobbler
Beverage(s)

DINNER
Baked Fish Buena
Vista
Mashed Potatoes
Broccoli, Buttered
Graham Rolls
Butter or Margarine
Banana Cream Pie
Beverage(s)

SUPPER
Cream of Celery
Soup
Sliced Cold Cuts
Jellied Cranberry
Salad
White and Dark Bread
Butter or Margarine
Baked Rice Custard
Beverage(s)

SUPPER
New England Clam
Chowder
Macaroni and Cheese

Jellied Pineapple and
Carrot Salad
Rolls
Butter or Margarine
Oatmeal Drop
Cookies
Beverage(s)

· SATURDAY

BREAKFAST
   Assorted Juices
   Buttermilk Pancakes
   Honey Butter
   Warm Maple Syrup
   Grilled Ham
   Beverage(s)

DINNER
   Goulash and Buttered
      Noodles
   Vegetable and Egg
      Salad
   Bread, white and dark
   Butter or Margarine
   Chilled Peaches
   Beverage(s)

SUPPER
   Cream of Vegetable
      Soup
   Cheeseburger
   Potato Chips
   Whole Kernel Corn
   Lemon Refrigerator
      Dessert
   Beverage(s)

8th Week

SUNDAY	MONDAY

BREAKFAST
 Chilled Orange Juice
 Country Fresh Eggs
 Grilled Sausages
 Almond Nut
  Doughnuts
 Butter or Margarine
 Beverage(s)

BREAKFAST
 Fruit in Season
 Old Fashioned Waffles
 Crisp Bacon
 Honey or Maple Syrup
 Soft Butter
 Beverage(s)

DINNER
 Chicken Chow Mein
  with Chinese
  Noodles
 Buttered Rice
 Mixed Salad Greens/
  Dressing
 Sesame Rolls
 Butter or Margarine
 Ice Cream—Fortune
  Cookies

DINNER
 Salisbury Steak
 Parsley on Buttered
  Potatoes
 Carrot Coins
 Molded Lime and
  Pear Salad
 Rolls
 Butter or Margarine
 Prune Cake
 Beverage(s)

SUPPER
 Split Pea Soup
 Sliced Ham Sand-
  wiches on ½ black
  and ½ white bread
 Hot Potato Salad

 Relishes
 Chilled Pineapple
  Chunks
 Beverage(s)

SUPPER
 Cream of Corn Soup
 Pimiento Cheese Sand-
  wiches
 Buttered Green Beans
 Apple, Celery, Tokay
  Grape Salad
 Pineapple Cream
  Pudding
 Beverage(s)

TUESDAY

BREAKFAST
   Assorted Juice
   Poached Egg on
      Buttered Toast
   Orange Pineapple
      Danish Roll
   Butter or Margarine
   Jelly
   Beverage(s)

DINNER
   Ham Loaf
   Mashed Sweet Potatoes
   Buttered Asparagus
   Tossed Green Salad/
      Dressing
   Bread, white and dark
   Butter or Margarine
   Old Fashioned Bread
      Pudding with Cust-
      ard Sauce
   Beverage(s)

SUPPER
   French Onion Soup

   Hot Beef Sandwich
   French Fried Potatoes
   Boiled Lima Beans
   Carrot and Raisin
      Salad
   Orange Cake
   Beverage(s)

WEDNESDAY

BREAKFAST
   Half Grapefruit
   Selected Cold Cereal
      or
   Wheatena, with Cream
   Golden Toast
   Butter or Margarine
   Jelly
   Beverage(s)

DINNER
   Beef Vegetable Soup
   Meat Loaf
   Browned Potatoes
   Buttered Carrots
   Red Cabbage and
      Apple Salad
   Chocolate Brownies

   Beverage(s)

SUPPER
   Chicken Rice Soup
   Bacon and Peanut
      Butter Sand-
      wich and
   Roast Beef
      Sandwiches
   Fruit Salad
   Oatmeal Crispies
      Cookies
   Beverage(s)

THURSDAY	FRIDAY

BREAKFAST
  Chilled Fruit Juice
  Buttermilk Pancakes
  Soft Butter
  Warm Maple Syrup
    or Honey
  Beverage(s)

BREAKFAST
  Orange Slices
  Scrambled Eggs
  Crisp Bacon
  Toast
  Butter or Margarine
  Jelly
  Beverage(s)

DINNER
  Liver and Bacon
  Buttered Potatoes
  Baked Onions with
    Tomatoes
  Jellied Vegetable
    Salad
  Apricot Upside-
    Down Cake
  Beverage(s)

DINNER
  Tuna Fish a la King
  served on Corn
    Bread
  Buttered Peas
  Jellied Tomato
    Salad
  Chilled Pears
  Beverage(s)

SUPPER
  Cream of Mushroom
    Soup
  Ham Salad and Egg
    Salad Sandwiches
  Bowl Salad
  Cinnamon Drop
    Cookies
  Beverage(s)

SUPPER
  Mulligatawny Soup

  French Toast
  Warm Maple Syrup
  Pineapple Cottage
    Cheese Salad
  Stewed Dried Peaches
  Beverage(s)

SATURDAY

BREAKFAST
Stewed Prunes,
    Lemon Slices
Assorted Cold Cereals
            or
Oatmeal, with Cream
Apple Streusel Danish
Butter or Margarine
Beverage(s)

DINNER
Baked Spareribs
    and Sauerkraut
Boiled Potatoes
Bread, white and dark
Butter or Margarine
Ice Cream, Cookies
Beverage(s)

SUPPER
Apple Cider
Turkey Salad
Rolls
Butter or Margarine
Baked Rice Custard
Beverage(s)

9th Week

SUNDAY

BREAKFAST
Grapefruit and
  Orange Sections
Bacon Omelet
Golden Toast
Butter or Margarine
Jam or Marmalade
Beverage(s)

DINNER
Oven Fried Golden
  Brown Chicken
Mashed Potatoes
Buttered Green Peas
Royal Orange and
  Apple Salad
Rolls
Butter or Margarine
Apricot Whip
Beverage(s)

SUPPER
Puree of Lima
  Bean Soup
Denver Egg Sandwich
Tomatoes with Celery
Tossed Vegetable
  Salad
Blueberry Cobbler
Beverage(s)

MONDAY

BREAKFAST
Chilled Fruit Juice
Assorted Cold Cereals
  or
Wheatena, with Cream
Apricot Danish Roll
Butter or Margarine
Beverage(s)

DINNER
Veal Scallopine
Buttered Noodles
Buttered Broccoli
Rolls
Butter or Margarine
Vanilla Ice Cream—
  Cookies
Beverage(s)

SUPPER
Chicken Rice Soup
Potato Pancakes
Applesauce, warm
Butterscotch Pudding
Beverage(s)

TUESDAY	WEDNESDAY

BREAKFAST
  Stewed Apricots
  Fried Egg
  Hickory Smoked
    Bacon
  Golden Toast
  Butter or Margarine
  Jam
  Beverage(s)

DINNER
  New England Boiled
    Dinner
    (including potatoes,
    carrots, onions,
    cabbage)
  Sliced Tomato on
    Lettuce
  Rolls
  Butter or Margarine
  Angel Food Cake
  Beverage(s)

SUPPER
  Cream of Mushroom
    Soup
  Welsh Rarebit on
    Toast (Cheese)

  Tossed Green Salad

  Sliced Pineapple—
    Cookies
  Beverage(s)

BREAKFAST
  Chilled Pineapple Juice
  Assorted Cold Cereals
    or
  Oatmeal, with cream
  Hot Rolls
  Butter or Margarine
  Jelly
  Beverage(s)

DINNER
  Broiled Lamb Patties
    on Grilled Pine-
    apple
  Delmonico Potatoes

  Rolls
  Butter or Margarine
  Jellied Cranberry
    Salad
  Lemon Refrigerator
    Dessert
  Beverage(s)

SUPPER
  Corn Chowder
  Ham and Pickle Sand-
    wich Filling on
    dark bread
  Buttered Green Beans
  Cherry Gelatin Cubes
  Beverage(s)

THURSDAY	FRIDAY
BREAKFAST	**BREAKFAST**
Grapefruit Sections, Grenadine	Chilled Prune Juice
Poached Egg on Buttered Toast	Old Fashioned Waffles
Apple Danish Roll	Honey Butter
Butter or Margarine	Warm Maple Syrup
Beverage(s)	Beverage(s)

THURSDAY

BREAKFAST
Grapefruit Sections,
  Grenadine
Poached Egg on
  Buttered Toast
Apple Danish Roll
Butter or Margarine
Beverage(s)

DINNER
Beef Stroganoff
  served with rice
Cucumber and Onion
  Salad
Roll
Butter or Margarine
Rainbow Sherbet
Beverage(s)

SUPPER
Pineapple Juice
Stuffed Peppers,
  Tomato Sauce
Orange-Apple Salad
  with Banana
Bread, white and dark
Butter or Margarine
Butterscotch Bars
Beverage(s)

FRIDAY

BREAKFAST
Chilled Prune Juice
Old Fashioned Waffles
Honey Butter
Warm Maple Syrup
Beverage(s)

DINNER
Macaroni and Cheese

Julienne Green Beans
Chopped Green
  Salad
Rolls
Butter or Margarine
Fruited Oatmeal Drop
  Cookies
Beverage(s)

SUPPER
Cream of Celery
  Soup
Fish Sticks
French Fried Potatoes
Sliced Tomatoes and
  Lettuce Salad
Bread
Sausage(s)
Apricot Whip
Beverage(s)

SATURDAY

BREAKFAST
   Chilled Fresh Melon
      Slice
   Assorted Cold Cereals
      ·   or
   Cream of Wheat,
      warm milk
   Cinnamon Coffeecake,
      butter or margarine
   Beverage(s)

DINNER
   Hungarian Goulash on
      Poppy Seed Noodles

   Bread, white and dark,
      also Crackers
   Butter or Margarine
   Jellied Pineapple and
      Carrot salad
   Lemon Pie
   Beverage(s)

SUPPER
   Scotch Broth
   Baked Frankfurters
      and Rice
   Marinated Bean Salad

   Southern Corn Muffins

   Cherry Gelatin/whipped
      topping
   Beverage(s)

10th Week

SUNDAY	MONDAY

BREAKFAST
  Chilled Melon
  Scrambled Eggs
  Hickory Smoked
    Bacon
  Corn Muffin
  Beverage(s)

BREAKFAST
  Assorted Fruit Juices
  Selected Cold Cereals
    or
  Oatmeal, with Cream
  Toast, Buttered
  Beverage(s)

DINNER
  Cranberry Juice
  Roast Pork
  Glazed Sweet
    Potatoes
  Pickled Crab Apples
  Three-Bean Vegetable
    Salad
  Pineapple Upside
    Down Cake/
    Topping
  Beverage(s)

DINNER
  Baked Beef Hash
  Buttered Spinach
  Tossed Green Salad/
    Dressing
  Rolls
  Butter or Margarine
  Mocha Nut Cake
  Beverage(s)

SUPPER
  Corn Chowder
  Ham Salad Sandwich
  Sliced Tomato and
    Lettuce
  Ice Cream and Raisin
    Cookies
  Beverage(s)

SUPPER
  Creamy Potato Soup

  Beef Macaroni Salad

  Deviled Eggs
  Hermit Cookies
  Beverage(s)

TUESDAY	**WEDNESDAY**

BREAKFAST
Orange Sections
Poached Egg on
   Buttered Toast

Hot Rolls
Butter or Margarine
Jam
Beverage(s)

DINNER
Barbecued Spare Ribs,
   with Sauce
Baked Potatoes, with
   butter
Green Beans, Julienne
Tossed Green Salad

Roll, wholewheat
Butter or Margarine
Chocolate Drop
   Cookies
Beverage(s)

SUPPER
Pork Chop Suey
   with Rice
Sunshine Salad
Rolls
Butter or Margarine
Baked Apple
Beverage(s)

BREAKFAST
Bananas with Cream
Golden French Toast
Maple Syrup or Honey
Canadian Bacon
Beverage(s)

DINNER
Scalloped Ham with
   Potatoes
Buttered Peas and
   Carrots
Pineapple Slaw
Rolls
Butter or Margarine
Prune Cake
Beverage(s)

SUPPER
Spaghetti with Tomato
   Meat Sauce
Buttered Broccoli
Bread, white and dark
Butter or Margarine
Chilled Pears
Beverage(s)

THURSDAY	FRIDAY

BREAKFAST
- Assorted Juices
- Selected Cold Cereal
  - or
- Wheatena, with Cream
- Apple Muffins
- Butter or Margarine
- Jelly
- Beverage(s)

BREAKFAST
- Grapefruit Half
- Fried Eggs
- Plantation Sausage
- Toast
- Butter or Margarine
- Jam
- Beverage(s)

DINNER
- Salisbury Steak
- Hashed Brown
  - Potatoes
- Buttered Cauliflower
- Jellied Pineapple and
  - Carrot Salad/
  - dressing
- Rolls
- Butter or Margarine
- Apple Brown Betty
- Beverage(s)

DINNER
- Salmon Loaf
- Au Gratin Potatoes

- Buttered Peas
- Tomato Aspic
- Rolls
- Butter or Margarine
- Apricot Tapioca
- Beverage(s)

SUPPER
- Cream of Vegetable
  - Soup
- Chicken and Noodle
  - Casserole
- Buttered Asparagus
- Whipped Grape Gelatin
- Beverage(s)

SUPPER
- Cream of Mushroom
  - Soup
- Welsh or Cheese Rarebit

- Pickles–Celery
- Buttered Carrots
- Purple Plums–Cookies
- Beverage(s)

SATURDAY

BREAKFAST
Assorted Juices
Buttermilk Pancakes
Honey Butter
Warm Maple Syrup
Grilled Ham
Beverage(s)

DINNER
Apple Juice
Burgundy Beef Stew

Buttered Spinach
Bread, white and dark
Butter or Margarine
Lemon Coconut Cake
Beverage(s)

SUPPER
French Onion Soup
Hamburger on Bun
    (barbecued)
French Fried Potatoes
Pineapple and Grated
    Cheese Salad
Grapenut Custard
    Pudding
Beverage(s)

11th Week

SUNDAY	MONDAY

BREAKFAST
Chilled Orange Juice
Country Fresh Eggs
Grilled Sausages
Sugar Doughnuts
Beverage(s)

BREAKFAST
Fruit in Season
Old Fashioned Waffles
Crisp Bacon
Honey or Maple Syrup
Soft Butter
Beverage(s)

DINNER
Fried Chicken
Whipped Potatoes
Corn, cream style
Carrot and Raisin
  Salad
Rolls
Butter or Margarine
Chocolate Cream Pie
Beverage(s)

DINNER
Swiss Steak
Hashed Brown
  Potatoes
Buttered Green Peas
Sunshine Salad
Bread
Butter or Margarine
Chilled Pears
Beverage(s)

SUPPER
Cream of Pea Soup
Large Fruit Salad
  (main dish)
Corn Muffins, warm

Butter or Margarine
Almond Nut Cookies
Beverage(s)

SUPPER
Celery Soup
Turkey or Chicken
  Spread Sandwiches
Escalloped Tomatoes
Butterscotch Ice Box
  Cookies
Beverage(s)

TUESDAY	WEDNESDAY

BREAKFAST
Assorted Juices
Poached Egg on
   Buttered Toast
Orange Pineapple
   Danish Roll
Butter or Margarine
Jelly
Beverage(s)

BREAKFAST
Half Grapefruit
Selected Cold Cereal
   or
Cream of Wheat, with
   cream
Golden Toast
Butter or Margarine
Jelly
Beverage(s)

DINNER
Beef Vegetable Stew

Asparagus
Pineapple and Cottage
   Cheese Salad
Bread
Butter or Margarine
Crumb Spice Cake
Beverage(s)

DINNER
Oven Baked Veal Chops
   and Gravy
Boiled Potatoes
Buttered Spinach
Raw Carrot and Raisin
   Salad
Butterscotch Pudding
Beverage(s)

SUPPER
Onion Tomato Soup
Chicken Pot Pie
Lettuce Salad –
   Dressing
Date Bars
Beverage(s)

SUPPER
Tomato-Rice Bouillon

Baked Macaroni and
   Cheese
Buttered Broccoli
Prune Crunch
Beverage(s)

THURSDAY	FRIDAY

BREAKFAST
Chilled Fruit Juice
Buttermilk Pancakes
Soft Butter
Warm Maple Syrup
   or Honey
Beverage(s)

BREAKFAST
Orange Slices
Scrambled Eggs
Crisp Bacon
Toast
Butter or Margarine
Jelly
Beverage(s)

DINNER
Grilled Liver and
   Bacon
Creamed Potatoes
   and Parsley
Buttered Whole Beets
Rolls
Butter or Margarine
Baked Custard
Beverage(s)

DINNER
Oven Fried Ocean
   Perch Fillets
Baked Potatoes
Stewed Tomatoes
   and Celery
Cabbage with Tart
   Sauce
Rolls
Butter or Margarine
Baked Apple
Beverage(s)

SUPPER
Swedish Rice Soup
Ham Salad and Egg
   Salad Sandwiches
Relishes
Apricot-Prune Pie
Beverage(s)

SUPPER
Beef Barley Soup
Creamed Codfish and
   Hard Cooked Eggs
   on Toast
Whipped Cherry Gelatin,
   Topping
Beverage(s)

SATURDAY

BREAKFAST
   Stewed Prunes, Lemon
      Slices
   Assorted Cold Cereals
            or
   Oatmeal, with Cream
   Blueberry Muffin
   Butter or Margarine
   Beverage(s)

DINNER
   Baked Ham
      Raisin Sauce
   Hot German Potato
      Salad
   Asparagus, Buttered
   Lettuce or Mixed Green
      Salad/Dressing
   Bread, white and dark
   Butter or Margarine
   Chilled Queen Anne
      Cherries
   Beverage(s)

SUPPER
   Bean Soup
   Spanish Rice with Meat
   Rolls
   Butter or Margarine
   Caramel Pudding
   Beverage(s)

12th Week

SUNDAY

BREAKFAST
    Grapefruit and
        Orange Sections
    Bacon Omelet
    Golden Toast
    Butter or Margarine
    Jam or Marmalade
    Beverage(s)

DINNER
    Roast Beef and
        Gravy
    Browned Potatoes
    Harvard Beets
    Chopped Cabbage and
        Raisin Slaw
    Rolls
    Butter or Margarine
    Honey Apple Pie
    Beverage(s)

SUPPER
    Chilled V-8 Juice
    Cold Plate, (Cheese,
        Ham, Roast Beef)
    Cottage Cheese
    Bread, white and dark
    Butter or Margarine
    Golden Chiffon
        Cake
    Beverage(s)

MONDAY

BREAKFAST
    Chilled Fruit Juice
    Assorted Cold Cereals
        or
    Wheatena, with Cream
    Cheese Danish Roll
    Butter or Margarine
    Beverage(s)

DINNER
    Breaded Veal
    Potatoes au Gratin
    Buttered Lima Beans
    Chopped Raw Salad
    Rolls
    Butter or Margarine
    Whipped Fruit Gelatin
    Beverage(s)

SUPPER
    Chicken Rice Soup

    Baked Green Peppers
        stuffed with Ground
        Meat and Tomato
        Sauce
    Cider Fruit Salad
    Bread, white and dark
    Butter or Margarine
    Brownies
    Beverage(s)

TUESDAY	WEDNESDAY

BREAKFAST
Stewed Apricots
Fried Egg
Hickory Smoked
  Bacon
Golden Toast
Butter or Margarine
Jam
Beverage(s)

DINNER
Meat Balls   in
  Mushroom Sauce

Parsley Buttered
  Potatoes
Tomatoes and Celery
Tossed Vegetable
  Salad/dressing
Rolls
Butter or Margarine
Banana Cake
Beverage(s)

SUPPER
Vegetable Soup
Fricassee of Chicken

Buttered Rice
Carrot and Raisin Salad

Whipped Red Rasp-
  berry gelatin,
  topping
Beverage(s)

BREAKFAST
Chilled Pineapple Juice
Assorted Cold Cereals
  or
Oatmeal, with Cream
Hot Rolls
Butter or Margarine
Jelly
Beverage(s)

DINNER
Veal Loaf
French Fried Potatoes
Cauliflower, creamed
Chef's Salad, Thousand
  Island Dressing
Rolls
Butter or Margarine
Cherry Nut Cookies
Beverage(s)

SUPPER
Rice and Tomato Soup

Corned Beef Sandwich
  or Egg Salad
  Sandwich
Succotash
Pineapple and Celery
  in Apple Gelatin
Banana Pudding
Beverage(s)

THURSDAY

BREAKFAST
  Grapefruit Sections
    Grenadine
  Poached Egg on
    Buttered Toast
  Apple Danish Roll
  Butter or Margarine
  Beverage(s)

DINNER
  Hungarian Goulash
    Poppyseed Noodles

  Buttered Asparagus
  Apricot-Raisin-Marsh-
    mallow Salad
  Wholewheat Rolls
  Butter or Margarine
  Caramel Custard
  Beverage(s)

SUPPER
  Beef Vegetable Soup
  American Pizza
  Spring Salad Bowl/
    dressing
  Coconut Cake
  Beverage(s)

FRIDAY

BREAKFAST
  Chilled Prune Juice
  Old Fashioned Waffles
  Honey Butter
  Warm Maple Syrup
  Beverage(s)

DINNER
  Fish Baked in White
    Wine
  Buttered Potatoes
    with Parsley
  Broccoli Spears
  Tomato Aspic
  Bread, white and dark
  Butter or Margarine
  Pineapple Chunks,
    chilled
  Beverage(s)

SUPPER
  V-8 Juice
  Salmon Salad
  Potato Chips
  Cottage Cheese with
    Chopped Spinach
  Graham Rolls
  Butter or Margarine
  Grape-Nut Custard
    Pudding
  Beverage(s)

SATURDAY

BREAKFAST
    Chilled Fresh Melon
        Slice
    Assorted Cold Cereals
            or
    Cream of Wheat,
        warm milk
    Cherry Coffeecake
    Butter or Margarine
    Beverage(s)

DINNER
    Apple Juice
    Turkey Macaroni Casserole
    Buttered Carrots and Peas
    Waldorf Salad
    Bread, white and dark
    Butter or Margarine, jelly
    Coconut Pineapple Squares
        (cookies)
    Beverage(s)

SUPPER
    Chicken Gumbo Soup

    Frankfurters and Sauer-
        kraut
    Black Bread
    Butter or Margarine
    German Potato Salad
    Mustard, Horseradish, Catsup
    Whipped Fruit Gelatin
    Beverage(s)

13th Week

SUNDAY

BREAKFAST
Chilled Melon
Scrambled Eggs
Hickory Smoked
Bacon
Cinnamon Raisin
Pecan Rolls
Beverage(s)

DINNER
Pork Roast
Whipped Sweet
Potatoes
Red Cinnamon
Apples
Buttered Peas
Pineapple and Carrot
in Gelatin Salad
Blueberry Muffins
Butter or Margarine
Lemon Refrigerator
Dessert
Beverage(s)

SUPPER
Cream of Celery Soup

Cold Plate (Pork, Cheese,
Ham, Potato Salad)
Bread, white and dark
Catsup
Cherry Tapioca—
Cookies
Beverage(s)

MONDAY

BREAKFAST
Assorted Fruit Juices
Selected Cold Cereals
or
Oatmeal, with Cream
Toast, Buttered
Jelly
Beverage(s)

DINNER
New England Boiled
Dinner (includes
potatoes)
Jellied Tomato Salad
Corn Bread
Butter, Margarine, Syrup
Stewed Apricots
Beverage(s)

SUPPER
V-8 Juice
Liver and Bacon
French Fried Potatoes
Buttered Broccoli
Rolls
Butter or Margarine
Peach Chiffon Dessert
Beverage(s)

TUESDAY

BREAKFAST
Orange Sections
Poached Egg on
   Buttered Toast
Hot Rolls
Butter or Margarine
Jam
Beverage(s)

DINNER
Turkey   and
   Dressing   and
   Giblet Gravy
Mashed Potatoes
Brussel Sprouts,
   buttered
Carrots, buttered
Jellied Orange and
   Cranberry Sauce
Rolls
Butter or Margarine
Baked Meringue Kisses

Beverage(s)

SUPPER
Turkey Soup
Open-faced Cheese
   and Tomato
   Sandwich, grilled
Chopped Cabbage Slaw

Whipped Raspberry
   Gelatin—cookies
Beverage(s)

WEDNESDAY

BREAKFAST
Bananas with Cream
Golden French Toast
Maple Syrup or Honey
Canadian Bacon
Beverage(s)

DINNER
Baked Beef Hash with
   Potatoes
Jullienne Green Beans
Jellied Royal Orange
   and Apple Salad
Rolls
Butter or Margarine
Baked Custard
Beverage(s)

SUPPER
Cream of Vegetable
   Soup
Corn Fritters
Crisp Bacon
Warm Maple Syrup
Stuffed Celery Sticks
   with American
   Cheddar Cheese
Fresh Fruits—selection
   of Bananas, Apples,
   Tangerines, Grapes
Beverage(s)

THURSDAY	FRIDAY

BREAKFAST
- Assorted Juices
- Selected Cold Cereal
  - or
- Wheatena, with Cream
- Corn Muffins
- Butter or Margarine
- Jelly
- Beverage(s)

BREAKFAST
- Grapefruit Half
- Fried Egg
- Plantation Sausage
- Toast
- Butter or Margarine
- Jam
- Beverage(s)

DINNER
- Veal Roast
- Baked, Buttered Squash
  with brown sugar
- Browned Potatoes
- Lettuce or Mixed Green
  Salad/Parisian dressing
- Hard Rolls
- Butter or Margarine
- Honey Apple Pie
- Beverage(s)

DINNER
- Baked Fish Buena Vista
- Buttered Parsley Potatoes
- Carrots, buttered
- Molded Perfection Salad

- Rolls
- Butter or Margarine
- Orange and Raisin
  Cupcakes
- Beverage(s)

SUPPER
- Apple Juice
- Chicken a la King
- Fresh Frozen Peas
- Royal Orange and
  Apple Salad
- Bread, white and dark
- Butter or Margarine
- Peanut Crunch Cookies

- Beverage(s)

SUPPER
- Tomato Rice Bouillon

- Cheese Fondue
- Buttered Cauliflower
- Jellied Beet Salad
- Rolls
- Butter or Margarine
- Pineapple Chiffon
  Pie
- Beverage(s)

SATURDAY

BREAKFAST
Assorted Juices
Buttermilk Pancakes
Honey Butter
Warm Maple Syrup
Grilled Ham
Beverage(s)

DINNER
Salisbury Steak
Scalloped Potatoes
Buttered Lima Beans
Head Lettuce, Vinegar
and Oil Dressing
Bread, white and dark
Butter or Margarine
Baked Rice Custard
Beverage(s)

SUPPER
Baked Lasagna
Tossed Green Salad/
Dressing
French Bread
Butter or Margarine
Blackberry Cobbler
Beverage(s)

14th Week

SUNDAY	MONDAY

BREAKFAST
    Chilled Orange Juice
    Country Fresh Egg
    Grilled Sausages
    Almond Nut Dough-
      nuts
    Butter or Margarine
    Beverage(s)

BREAKFAST
    Fruit in Season
    Old Fashioned Waffles
    Crisp Bacon
    Honey or Maple Syrup
    Soft Butter
    Beverage(s)

DINNER
    Roast Turkey
    Mashed Potatoes
    Zucchini and Tomatoes
    Asparagus
    Rolls
    Butter or Margarine
    Jellied Cranberry Salad
    Brownies
    Beverage(s)

DINNER
    Apple Cider
    Braised Pork Chops
    Glazed Sweet
      Potatoes
    Sliced Buttered Carrots
    Orange-Apple-Banana
      Salad
    Rolls
    Butter or Margarine
    Chilled Peaches
    Beverage(s)

SUPPER
    Beef Noodle Soup
    Cold Plate (Beef, Ham,
      Cheese Cuts)
    Buttered Carrots
    Bread, white and dark
    Butter or Margarine
    Vanilla Ice Cream,
      Cookies
    Beverage(s)

SUPPER
    Vegetable Soup
    Frankfurter and Roll
      (buttered)
    Catsup
    Boston Baked Beans
    Perfection Salad
      Squares
    Butterscotch Ice Box
      Cookies
    Beverage(s)

TUESDAY

BREAKFAST
  Assorted Juices
  Poached Egg on
    Buttered Toast
  Apricot Danish Roll
  Butter or Margarine
  Jelly
  Beverage(s)

DINNER
  Oven Fried Chicken

  Whipped Potatoes
    and Gravy
  Creamed Spinach
    with Onion and
    Crunchy Bacon
  Buttered Peas
  Sliced Tomato and
    Lettuce Salad
  Rolls, wholewheat
  Butter or Margarine
  Cubed Chilled Pine-
    apple
  Beverage(s)

SUPPER
  Bean Soup
  Minced Ham Sandwich
  Tossed Green Salad

  Fig-Nut Tapioca (nuts
    should be ground)
  Beverage(s)

WEDNESDAY

BREAKFAST
  Half Grapefruit
  Selected Cold Cereal
    or
  Cream of Wheat,
    with cream
  Golden Toast
  Butter or Margarine
  Jelly
  Beverage(s)

DINNER
  Barbecued Spare
    Ribs
  Boiled Potatoes
  Buttered Brussel
    Sprouts
  Bread, white and dark
  Butter or Margarine
  Watercress/French
    Dressing
  Angel Food Cake
  Beverage(s)

SUPPER
  Split Pea Soup
  Swedish Meat Balls,
    Buttered Rice
  Cooked Vegetable Salad,

  Chocolate Pudding,
    Whipped Cream
  Beverage(s)

THURSDAY	FRIDAY

BREAKFAST
- Chilled Fruit Juice
- Buttermilk Pancakes
- Soft Butter
- Warm Maple Syrup
  or Honey
- Beverage(s)

BREAKFAST
- Orange Slices
- Scrambled Eggs
- Crisp Bacon
- Toast
- Butter or Margarine
- Jelly
- Beverage(s)

DINNER
- Liver Creole
- Baked Potatoes
- Buttered Asparagus
- Jellied Pineapple and
  Carrot Salad
- Baking Powder
  Biscuits
- Butter or Margarine,
  Jam
- Chilled Pear Halves
- Beverage(s)

DINNER
- Shrimp and Crabmeat
  Newburg
- French Fried Potatoes
- Harvard Beets
- Tossed Salad
- Bread, white and dark
- Butter or Margarine
- Jelly Roll
- Beverage(s)

SUPPER
- Lima Bean Soup
- Swiss Steak
- Carrots and Peas
- Warm Apple Sauce
- Bread, white and dark
- Butter or Margarine
- Peanut Butter Cake
- Beverage(s)

SUPPER
- Cream of Tomato Soup

- Pancakes
- Warm Butter or
  Margarine
- Warm Maple Syrup
- Fresh Fruits (selection
  of Apples, Oranges,
  Bananas, Grapes)
- Beverage(s)

SATURDAY

BREAKFAST
  Stewed Prunes,
    Lemon Slices
  Assorted Cold Cereals
    or
  Oatmeal, with Cream
  Assorted Danish
  Butter or Margarine
  Beverage(s)

DINNER
  Swiss Steak
    (includes onions and
    tomatoes)
  Hashed Brown
    Potatoes
  Chopped Spinach with
    Bacon Dressing
  German Cucumber Salad
  Butterscotch Bars
  Beverage(s)

SUPPER
  Onion Soup
  Shepherd's Pie
  Royal Lime and
    Apple Salad
  Apricot Whip
  Beverage(s)

15th Week

SUNDAY	MONDAY

BREAKFAST
  Grapefruit and
    Orange Sections
  Bacon Omelet
  Golden Toast
  Butter or Margarine
  Jam or Marmalade
  Beverage(s)

BREAKFAST
  Chilled Fruit Juice
  Assorted Cold Cereals
    or
  Wheatena, with Cream
  Cheese Danish Roll
  Butter or Margarine
  Beverage(s)

DINNER
  Chicken Roasted
    with Stuffing
    and Giblet Gravy

  Baked Hubbard Squash

  Green Beans, French
    Style
  Jellied Cranberry and
    Orange Salad
  Rolls
  Butter or Margarine
  Blueberry Pie
  Beverage(s)

DINNER
  Baked Ham
  Potatoes au Gratin
  Buttered Lima Beans
  Bread, white and dark
  Butter or Margarine
  Head Lettuce, Roquefort
    Dressing
  Cherry Tapioca
  Beverage(s)

SUPPER
  Beef Rice Soup
  Cold Plate (Ham,
    Cheese, Sausage Loaf,
    Pickles and Olives)
  Potato Chips
  Bread, white and dark
  Butter or Margarine
  Lemon Coconut Cake
  Beverage(s)

SUPPER
  Baked Green Peppers,
    Stuffed with Ground
    Meat and Tomato
    Sauce
  Cider-Fruit Salad
  Rolls, Graham
  Butter or Margarine
  Brownies
  Beverage(s)

TUESDAY	WEDNESDAY

BREAKFAST
Stewed Apricots
Fried Egg
Hickory Smoked
  Bacon
Golden Toast
Butter or Margarine
Jam
Beverage(s)

BREAKFAST
Chilled Pineapple Juice
Assorted Cold Cereals
  or
Oatmeal, with Cream
Hot Rolls
Butter or Margarine
Jelly
Beverage(s)

DINNER
Liver and Bacon

Buttered Parsley
  Potatoes
Mixed Vegetables
Carrot-Apple-Raisin
  Salad
Rolls
Butter or Margarine
Baked Peach Halves
Beverage(s)

DINNER
Fried Veal Chops
  and Gravy
Boiled Potatoes
Buttered Chopped
  Spinach
Cole Slaw
Rolls
Butter or Margarine
Charlotte Russe
  (gelatin)
Beverage(s)

SUPPER
Corn Chowder
Stuffed Beef and
  Cabbage Rolls
Tomato Aspic
Pineapple Upside
  Down Cake
Beverage(s)

SUPPER
Beef Vegetable Soup
Meat and Cheese
  Salad Plate
Succotash
Pineapple and
  Lettuce Salad
Bread, white and dark
Butter or Margarine
Apple Turnovers
Beverage(s)

THURSDAY	FRIDAY
BREAKFAST Grapefruit Sections, 　Grenadine Poached Egg on 　Buttered Toast Apple Danish Roll Butter or Margarine Beverage(s)	**BREAKFAST** 　Chilled Prune Juice 　Old Fashioned Waffles 　Honey Butter 　Warm Maple Syrup 　Beverage(s)
DINNER 　Breaded Pork Chops, 　　Cream Gravy 　Boiled Potatoes 　Carrots and Peas 　Jellied Cranberries on 　　Lettuce 　Rolls 　Butter or Margarine 　Apple Pie 　Beverage(s)	**DINNER** 　Filet of Sole, 　　Tartar Sauce 　French Fried Potatoes 　Buttered, Sliced Carrots 　Red Cabbage and 　　Apple Salad 　Rolls 　Butter or Margarine 　Cream Pie 　Beverage(s)
SUPPER 　Boston Clam 　　Chowder 　Broiled Beef Patties 　Lettuce–Tomato 　　Salad/dressing 　Baked Potato 　Fruited Gelatin 　Beverage(s)	**SUPPER** 　Minestrone Soup and 　　Crackers 　Chicken Chow Mein, 　　Rice 　Beet and Egg Salad 　Fruit Whip 　Beverage(s)

SATURDAY

BREAKFAST
  Chilled Melon
    Slice
  Assorted Cold Cereals
        or
  Cream of Wheat,
    warm milk
  Cinnamon Raisin
    Pecan Roll
  Butter or Margarine
  Beverage(s)

DINNER
  Meat Balls
    Spaghetti Milani
  Green Beans, buttered
  Tossed Green Salad/
    dressing
  Rolls
  Butter or Margarine
  Applesauce Cake
  Beverage(s)

SUPPER
  French Onion Soup
  Tomato Stuffed with
    Chicken Salad
  Buttered Asparagus
  Corn Bread
  Butter or
    Margarine—Syrup
  Spice Cake with Frosting
  Beverage(s)

16th Week

SUNDAY	MONDAY

BREAKFAST
  Chilled Melon
  Scrambled Eggs
  Hickory Smoked
    Bacon
  Sugar Doughnuts
  Beverage(s)

DINNER
  Apple Juice
  Roast Turkey and
    Gravy
  Bread Stuffing
  Mashed Potatoes
  Buttered Mixed
    Vegetables
  Cranberry Sauce
  Nut Bread
  Butter or Margarine
  Ice Cream—Cookies
  Beverage(s)

SUPPER
  Tomato-Rice
    Bouillon
  Corned Beef Sand-
    wiches,
    Rye Bread
  Potato Chips
  Stuffed Celery Sticks
    and Carrot Sticks
  Apricot Whip
  Beverage(s)

BREAKFAST
  Assorted Fruit Juices
  Selected Cold Cereals
    or
  Oatmeal, with Cream
  Toast, buttered
  Jelly
  Beverage(s)

DINNER
  Baked Meat Loaf
  Browned Potatoes
  Lima Beans
  Cole Slaw
  Bread, white and dark
  Butter or Margarine
  Cherry Tapioca
  Beverage(s)

SUPPER
  Beef Noodle Soup
  Scalloped Egg Plant
    with Mushrooms
    on Toast
  Fresh Fruits (Apples,
    Bananas, Oranges,
    Grapes)
  Beverage(s)

TUESDAY	WEDNESDAY

BREAKFAST
  Orange Sections
  Poached Egg on
    Buttered Toast
  Hot Rolls
  Butter or Margarine
  Jam
  Beverage(s)

BREAKFAST
  Bananas with Cream
  Golden French Toast
  Maple Syrup or Honey
  Canadian Bacon
  Beverage(s)

DINNER
  Pot Roast of Beef,
    Natural Gravy
  Mashed Potatoes
  Beets with Orange
    Sauce
  Mixed Green Salad/
    dressing
  Bread, white and dark
  Butter or Margarine
  Bread Pudding with
    Vanilla Sauce
  Beverage(s)

DINNER
  Baked Virginia Ham
    Raisin Sauce
  Mashed Sweet Potatoes
  Stewed Tomatoes
    with Celery
  Spiced Peach Salad
  Bread, white and dark
  Butter or Margarine
  Lemon Cream Pie
  Beverage(s)

SUPPER
  Chicken Noodle
    Soup
  Sirloin Patties
  Buttered Wax Beans
  Cabbage and Green
    Pepper Salad
  Rolls
  Butter or Margarine
  Chilled Queen Anne
    Cherries
  Beverage(s)

SUPPER
  Onion Tomato Soup
  Grilled Frankfurter
  Hot Potato Salad
  Brown Bread
  Butter or Margarine
  Chilled Pears
  Beverage(s)

THURSDAY	FRIDAY

BREAKFAST
Assorted Juices
Selected Cold Cereal
or
Wheatena, with Cream
Corn Muffins
Butter or Margarine
Jelly
Beverage(s)

BREAKFAST
Grapefruit Half
Fried Egg
Plantation Sausage
Toast
Butter or Margarine
Jam
Beverage(s)

DINNER
City Chicken Legs
and Cream Gravy
Boiled Potatoes
Green Beans
Perfection Salad/
dressing
Bread
Butter or Margarine
Devils Food Cake
Beverage(s)

DINNER
Golden Tuna Casserole
Buttered Asparagus
Royal Orange and
Apple Salad
Rolls
Butter or Margarine
Stewed Dried Peaches
Beverage(s)

SUPPER
Split Pea Soup
Macaroni and Cheese
Casserole
Orange and Grapefruit
Salad
Bread, white or dark
Butter or Margarine
Raisin Cookies
Beverage(s)

SUPPER
Cream of Potato
Soup
Fruit Salad
Cottage Cheese
Corn Muffins
Butter or Margarine,
Jelly
Angel Food Cake /
Topping
Beverage(s)

SATURDAY

BREAKFAST
  Stewed Prunes
  Buttered Pancakes
  Honey Butter
  Warm Maple Syrup
  Grilled Ham
  Beverage(s)

DINNER
  Swiss Steak, gravy
  Mashed Potatoes
  Cut Green Beans,
    Buttered
  Tossed Green Salad
  Corn Bread
  Butter or Margarine,
    Syrup
  Orange Sherbet
  Beverage(s)

SUPPER
  Cream of Chicken Soup

  Hot Sliced Pork Roast
    and Gravy Sandwich
  Beet and Onion Salad
  Whipped Fruit Gelatin
  Beverage(s)

17th Week

SUNDAY

BREAKFAST
Chilled Orange Juice
Country Fresh Eggs
Grilled Sausages
Coconut Doughnuts

Beverage(s)

DINNER
Roast Beef au Jus

Mashed Potatoes
Buttered Cauliflower
Cloverleaf Rolls
Butter or Margarine
Cherry Cobbler
Beverage(s)

SUPPER
Apple Juice
Chicken Fricassee
Hot Biscuits
Pear and Cottage
Cheese on Romaine
with dressing
Butter or Margarine
Ginger Cookies
Beverage(s)

MONDAY

BREAKFAST
Fruit in Season
Old Fashioned Waffles
Crisp Bacon
Honey or Maple Syrup
Soft Butter
Beverage(s)

DINNER
Braised Beef with
Vegetables
Boiled Potatoes
Buttered Green Beans
Cabbage-Apple-Pine-
apple Salad
Rolls
Butter or Margarine
Vanilla Cream Pudding
Beverage(s)

SUPPER
Vegetable Soup
Egg Salad Sandwich
or Ham Sandwich
Jellied Fruit Salad
Prune Cookies
Beverage(s)

TUESDAY	WEDNESDAY

BREAKFAST
- Assorted Juices
- Poached Egg on
  - Buttered Toast
- Orange-Pineapple
  - Danish Roll
- Butter or Margarine
- Jelly
- Beverage(s)

BREAKFAST
- Half Grapefruit
- Selected Cold Cereal
  - or
- Cream of Wheat,
  - with Cream
- Golden Toast
- Butter or Margarine
- Jelly
- Beverage(s)

DINNER
- Breaded Veal
  - Cutlet
- Whipped Potatoes
- Creamed Spinach
- Rolls
- Butter or Margarine
- Gingerbread with
  - Lemon Sauce
- Beverage(s)

DINNER
- Roast Loin of Pork

- Mashed Yams
- Tossed Green Salad

- Beets with Orange
  - Sauce
- Rolls
- Butter or Margarine
- Devil's Food Cake

- Beverage(s)

SUPPER
- Chilled V-8 Juice
- Potato Pancakes
- Apple Sauce
- Mixed Green Salad/
  - dressing
- Chilled Pear Half
- Beverage(s)

SUPPER
- Veal Scallopini
- Buttered Cut Corn
- Corn Muffins
- Butter or Margarine
- Prune and Cottage
  - Cheese Salad
- Pineapple Cream
  - Pudding
- Beverage(s)

THURSDAY	FRIDAY

BREAKFAST
  Chilled Fruit Juice
  Buttermilk Pancakes
  Soft Butter
  Warm Maple Syrup
    or Honey
  Beverage(s)

BREAKFAST
  Orange Slices
  Scrambled Eggs
  Crisp Bacon
  Toast
  Butter or Margarine
  Jelly
  Beverage(s)

DINNER
  Beef Pot Roast
  Potatoes au Gratin
  Diced Buttered
    Turnips and Peas
  Orange and Grapefruit
    Sections Salad/
    dressing
  Rolls
  Butter or Margarine
  Butterscotch Custard
    Pie
  Beverage(s)

DINNER
  Oven Fried Ocean
    Perch Fillets
  Potato Puff
    (Duchess)
  Buttered Broccoli
    Spears
  Chopped Salad Greens/
    Russian Dressing
  Rolls
  Butter or Margarine
  Apple Pie
  Beverage(s)

SUPPER
  Minestrone Soup
  Weiner and Baked Beans
  Spinach
  Bread, white and dark
  Golden Chiffon Cake
    with Icing
  Beverage(s)

SUPPER
  Cream of Asparagus
    Soup
  Rice and Cheese Omelet
  Lima Beans
  Bread, white and dark
  Butter or Margarine
  Chilled Peaches
  Beverage(s)

SATURDAY

BREAKFAST
  Stewed Prunes,
    Lemon Slices
  Assorted Cold Cereals
      or
  Oatmeal, with Cream
  Cinnamon Streusel
    Danish
  Butter or Margarine
  Beverage(s)

DINNER
  Salisbury Steak, gravy
  Mashed Sweet Potatoes
  Buttered Peas
  Pan Rolls
  Butter or Margarine
  Cabbage and Ground
    Peanut Salad
  Pineapple Chunks,
    chilled
  Beverage(s)

SUPPER
  Potato and Onion
    Soup
  Barbecued Ground
    Beef on Bun
  Jellied Vegetable
    Salad
  Blueberry Cobbler
  Beverage(s)

18th Week

SUNDAY	MONDAY
BREAKFAST	**BREAKFAST**
Grapefruit and Orange Sections	Chilled Fruit Juice
Bacon Omelet	Assorted Cold Cereals
Golden Toast	or
Butter or Margarine	Wheatena, with Cream
Jam or Marmalade	Cheese Danish Roll
Beverage(s)	Butter or Margarine
	Beverage(s)

SUNDAY

BREAKFAST
Grapefruit and
    Orange Sections
Bacon Omelet
Golden Toast
Butter or Margarine
Jam or Marmalade
Beverage(s)

DINNER
Roast Leg of Lamb,
    Mint Jelly
Baked Potato
Buttered Broccoli
    Cuts
Assorted Pickles
Carrot and Pineapple
    Salad
Rolls
Butter or Margarine
Peach Pie
Beverage(s)

SUPPER
Tomato Bouillon

Spanish Rice with
    chopped meat
Bread—Butter or
    Margarine
Pear and Grated Cheese
    Salad/dressing
Grapenut Pudding
Beverage(s)

MONDAY

BREAKFAST
Chilled Fruit Juice
Assorted Cold Cereals
    or
Wheatena, with Cream
Cheese Danish Roll
Butter or Margarine
Beverage(s)

DINNER
Baked Veal Shoulder
    with Stuffing,
    Natural Gravy
Boiled Potatoes
Buttered Cauliflower
Lettuce Salad/
    dressing
Rolls
Butter or Margarine
Bread Pudding with
    Chocolate Sauce
Beverage(s)

SUPPER
Chicken-Pimiento Soup
Sliced Cold Meats
Hot Potato Salad
Assorted Pickles
Wholewheat Bread
Butter or Margarine
Fruit Cup
Beverage(s)

TUESDAY

BREAKFAST
Stewed Apricots
Fried Egg
Hickory Smoked
  Bacon
Golden Toast
Butter or Margarine
Jam
Beverage(s)

DINNER
Braised Chopped
  Beef Steaks
Creamed Potatoes
Buttered Corn and
  Green Peppers Saute
Shredded Cabbage and
  Carrot Salad
Rolls
Butter or Margarine
Brown Sugar Custard
Beverage(s)

SUPPER
Clam Chowder
Cheese Rarebit with
  Bacon
Baked Stuffed
  Tomatoes
Shredded Lettuce
  Salad
Whipped Fruit Gelatin
Beverage(s)

WEDNESDAY

BREAKFAST
Chilled Pineapple Juice
Assorted Cold Cereals
  or
Oatmeal, with Cream
Hot Rolls
Butter or Margarine
Jelly
Beverage(s)

DINNER
German Pot Roast
  (Sauerbraten)

Oven Browned Potatoes
Buttered Cut Green
  Beans
Vegetable Salad,
  Jellied
Rolls
Butter or Margarine
Gingerbread
  Topping
Beverage(s)

SUPPER
Cream of Spinach
  Soup
Barbecued Ham-
  burgers on Bun
Potato Chips
Carrot Sticks
Tapioca Pudding
Beverage(s)

THURSDAY	FRIDAY

BREAKFAST
Grapefruit Sections,
    Grenadine
Poached Egg on
    Buttered Toast
Apricot Danish Roll
Butter or Margarine
Beverage(s)

BREAKFAST
Chilled Prune Juice
Old Fashioned Waffles
Honey Butter
Warm Maple Syrup
Beverage(s)

DINNER
Ham with Potatoes
    au Gratin
Buttered Asparagus
Ginger Ale Fruit Salad/
    dressing
Bread, wholewheat
Butter or Margarine
Thick Molasses
    Cookies
Beverage(s)

DINNER
V-8 Juice
Scallops, deep fried
    with lemon
Lyonnaise Potatoes
Buttered Broccoli
Bread, white and dark
Butter or Margarine
Fruit Shortcake
Beverage(s)

SUPPER
Mushroom Soup
Chicken Salad
    Sandwiches
Tomato Aspic
Gold Pound Cake/
    Topping
Beverage(s)

SUPPER
Baked Macaroni and
    Cheese
Red Cabbage, German
    Style
Fruit Salad with Stuffed
    Prunes
Rolls
Butter or Margarine
Apple Pie
Beverage(s)

SATURDAY

BREAKFAST
  Chilled Fresh Melon Slice
  Assorted Cold Cereals
        or
  Cream of Wheat,
     warm milk
  Blueberry Muffin
  Butter or Margarine
  Beverage(s)

DINNER
  Beef and Pepper Steak
  Tossed Vegetable Salad

  Bread, wholewheat
  Butter or Margarine
  Cantaloupe, chilled
  Beverage(s)

SUPPER
  Vegetable Soup
  Chicken Chow Mein
     over Chinese Noodles
  Rice, mound
  Celery and String Bean
     Salad
  Yellow Cup Cakes/
     Frosting
  Beverage(s)

19th Week

SUNDAY

BREAKFAST
Chilled Melon
Scrambled Eggs
Hickory Smoked
  Bacon
Cinnamon Raisin
  Pecan Rolls
Beverage(s)

DINNER
Baked Meat Loaf
  with Gravy
Home Fried Potatoes

Glazed Carrot Slices

Peas, buttered
Three-Bean Salad
Rolls
Butter or Margarine
Vanilla Ice Cream—
  Butterscotch Sauce
Beverage(s)

SUPPER
Tomato Rice Soup

Chicken Pie
Yankee Slaw
Bread, white and dark
Butter or Margarine
Chilled Peaches—
  Cookies
Beverage(s)

MONDAY

BREAKFAST
Assorted Fruit Juices
Selected Cold Cereals
  or
Oatmeal, with Cream
Toast, with butter
Jelly
Beverage(s)

DINNER
Sirloin Tips, gravy
Shelled Macaroni
  Florentine
Broccoli, buttered
Pineapple and Rasp- •
  berry Gelatin Salad
Rolls
Butter or Margarine
Cottage Pudding with
  Lemon Sauce
Beverage(s)

SUPPER
Chicken Mushroom
  Soup
Ham and Potatoes au
  Gratin
Creamed Corn
Bread, white and dark
Butter or Margarine
Devils Food Cake
  Squares
Beverage(s)

TUESDAY	WEDNESDAY
BREAKFAST	**BREAKFAST**
Orange Sections	Bananas with Cream
Poached Egg on	Golden French Toast
Buttered Toast	Maple Syrup or Honey
Hot Rolls	Canadian Bacon
Butter or Margarine	Beverage(s)
Jam	
Beverage(s)	
DINNER	**DINNER**
Barbecued Short Ribs	Braised Minute Steaks
Oven Browned Potatoes	and Gravy
Buttered Spinach	Mashed Potatoes
Tossed Lettuce and	Green Buttered Beans
Orange Section	Stuffed Prune
Salad	Salad
Rolls	Roll, wholewheat
Butter or Margarine	Butter or Margarine
Lemon Fluff	Pineapple Upside
Beverage(s)	Down Cake
	Beverage(s)
SUPPER	**SUPPER**
Beef Soup with	Corn Chowder
Barley	Chicken Salad
Barbecued Meat Balls	Potato Chips
on Fluffy Rice	Relishes
Grated Carrot and	Bread, white and dark
Raisin Salad	Butter or Margarine
Baked Cherry	Rice Pudding
Pudding	Beverage(s)
Beverage(s)	

THURSDAY

BREAKFAST
Assorted Juices
Selected Cold Cereal
or
Wheatena, with Cream
Corn Muffins
Butter or Margarine
Jelly
Beverage(s)

DINNER
Roast Lamb and
Mint Jelly
Buttered Parsley
Potatoes
Fritter Fried Egg
Plant
Parker House Rolls

Butter or Margarine
Sliced Tomato Salad
Apricot Tapioca
Beverage(s)

SUPPER
Beef Bouillon
Creamed Egg Golden-
rod on Toast
Baby Lima Beans
Cream Puffs, Choco-
late Icing
Beverage(s)

FRIDAY

BREAKFAST
Grapefruit Half
Fried Egg
Plantation Sausage
Toast
Butter or Margarine
Jam
Beverage(s)

DINNER
Broiled Haddock
Delmonico Potatoes

Swiss Chard
Strawberry Aspic with
Cottage Cheese Layer
Rolls
Butter or Margarine
Banana Shortcake—
Topping
Beverage(s)

SUPPER
Cream of Asparagus
Soup
Tunafish Salad on
Lettuce Leaf
Potato Chips
Celery and Olives
Bread, wholewheat
Butter or Margarine
Honey Drop
Cookies
Beverage(s)

SATURDAY

BREAKFAST
  Assorted Juices
  Buttermilk Pancakes
  Honey Butter
  Warm Maple Syrup
  Grilled Ham
  Beverage(s)

DINNER
  Spare Ribs and
    Sauerkraut
  Boiled Potatoes
  Tomato Aspic
  Rolls
  Butter or Margarine
  Spice Cake/topping
  Beverage(s)

SUPPER
  Fried Vienna Sausages
  Spaghetti with Butter
    sauce
  Green Beans, buttered
  Tomato and Lettuce
    Salad
  Bread, white and dark
  Butter or Margarine
  Whipped Fruit Gelatin
  Beverage(s)

20th Week

SUNDAY

BREAKFAST
Chilled Orange Juice
Country Fresh Egg
Grilled Sausages
Chocolate Dough-
nuts
Butter or Margarine
Beverage(s)

DINNER
Creamed Chicken in
Individual Shells

Baked Potato, Sour
Cream and Chives
Asparagus and Pimiento
Tossed Salad (green)/
dressing
Rolls
Butter or Margarine
Orange-Cranberry Pie
Beverage(s)

SUPPER
Tomato Rice
Bouillon
Choice of Bologna,
Egg Salad and
Cheese Sandwiches
Relishes—Pickles
Catsup, Horseradish Mustard
Raw Vegetable Salad/
dressing
Apple Crisp
Beverage(s)

MONDAY

BREAKFAST
Fruit in Season
Old Fashioned Waffles
Crisp Bacon
Honey or Maple Syrup
Soft Butter
Beverage(s)

DINNER
Spanish Rice with Meat
Cauliflower with Buttered
Bread Crumbs
Pear Salad with Cream
Cheese
Rolls, wholewheat
Butter or Margarine
Fruit Pudding—Custard
Sauce
Beverage(s)

SUPPER
Cream of Celery Soup

Welsh Rarebit on Toast

Green Peas, buttered
Jellied Fruit Salad/
Cream Dressing
Oatmeal Date Bars
Beverage(s)

TUESDAY

BREAKFAST
  Assorted Juices
  Poached Egg on
    Buttered Toast
  Apricot Danish Roll
  Butter or Margarine
  Jelly
  Beverage(s)

DINNER
  Veal Breasts with
    Stuffing
  Buttered Parsley
    Potatoes
  Fried Egg Plant
  Lettuce and Tomato
    Salad
  Bread, white and dark
  Butter or Margarine
  Strawberry Chiffon
    Pie
  Beverage(s)

SUPPER
  Pork and Veal
    Chop Suey
  Chinese Noodles
  Buttered Rice
  Lime Pear Aspic

  Bread, white and dark
  Butter or Margarine
  Fluffy White Cake with
    Orange Frosting
  Beverage(s)

WEDNESDAY

BREAKFAST
  Half Grapefruit
  Selected Cold Cereal
    or
  Cream of Wheat,
    with Cream
  Golden Toast
  Butter or Margarine
  Jelly
  Beverage(s)

DINNER
  Grilled Liver and
    Bacon
  Buttered Parsley
    Potatoes
  Scalloped Tomatoes

  Watercress with
    French Dressing
  Bread, white and dark
  Butter or Margarine
  Chocolate Cottage
    Pudding with
    Custard Sauce
  Beverage(s)

SUPPER
  Cranberry Juice
  Ham and Sweet Potato
    Casserole
  Green Beans
  Bread, white and dark
  Butter or Margarine
  Whipped Gelatin with
    Topping
  Beverage(s)

THURSDAY	FRIDAY

BREAKFAST
Chilled Fruit Juice
Buttermilk Pancakes
Soft Butter
Warm Maple Syrup
    or Honey
Beverage(s)

BREAKFAST
Orange Slices
Scrambled Eggs
Crisp Bacon
Toast
Butter or Margarine
Jelly
Beverage(s)

DINNER
Braised Beef with
    Potatoes, Carrots,
    and Peas
Bread, white and dark
Butter or Margarine
Jellied Crushed Pine-
    apple in Lemon
    Gelatin Salad
Peach Cobbler
Beverage(s)

DINNER
Scallops and Shrimp
    Newburg with
    Green Peas
Potato Chips
Buttered Broccoli
    Spears
Rolls
Butter or Margarine
Grape Nut Custard
Beverage(s)

SUPPER
Beef Noodle Soup
Baked Green Pepper
    stuffed, Tomato
    sauce
Roll, wholewheat
Butter or Margarine
Chilled Queen Anne
    Cherries
Beverage(s)

SUPPER
Cream of Asparagus
    Soup
Salmon Loaf
Apple,Celery and
    Date Salad
Bread, white and dark
Butter or Margarine
Crispy Oatmeal
    Cookies
Beverage(s)

SATURDAY

BREAKFAST
    Stewed Prunes,
       Lemon Slices
    Assorted Cold Cereals
         or
    Oatmeal, with Cream
    Prune Danish
    Butter or Margarine
    Beverage(s)

DINNER
    Hamburger Steak
      with Fried Onions

    Buttered Noodles
    Cole Slaw
    Harvard Beets
    Rolls
    Butter or Margarine
    Brown Sugar Custard
    Beverage(s)

SUPPER
    Scotch Broth with
      Barley
    Shepherd's Pie,
      Whipped Potato
      Crust
    Bread, white and dark
    Butter or Margarine
    Pineapple Sherbet
    Beverage(s)

21st Week

SUNDAY	MONDAY
BREAKFAST	**BREAKFAST**

BREAKFAST
Grapefruit and Orange
    Sections
Bacon Omelet
Golden Toast
Butter or Margarine
Jam or Marmalade
Beverage(s)

DINNER
Roast Loin of
    Pork
Brown Gravy
Mashed Potatoes
Buttered Baby
    Lima Beans
Carrot and Raisin
    Salad
Hot Biscuits
Butter or Margarine
Lemon Pie
Beverage(s)

SUPPER
Tomato Barley
    Soup
½ Liverwurst Sand-
    wich (dark bread)
½ Deviled Egg Sand-
    wich (white bread)
Relishes
Potato Chips
Spice Cake with
    Whipped Cream
Beverage(s)

BREAKFAST
Chilled Fruit Juice
Assorted Cold Cereals
    or
Wheatena, with Cream
Lemon Doughnut
Beverage(s)

DINNER
Boiled Weiners with
    German Sauerkraut
Boiled Potatoes
Harvard Beets
Bread, white and dark
Butter or Margarine
Baked Rice Custard
Beverage(s)

SUPPER
Vegetable Soup,
    saltines
Broiled Cheeseburger
    on large Bun
Green Beans, buttered
Whipped Apple Gelatin
    with Bananas
Beverage(s)

TUESDAY

BREAKFAST
  Stewed Apricots
  Fried Egg
  Hickory Smoked
    Bacon
  Golden Toast
  Butter or Margarine
  Jam
  Beverage(s)

DINNER
  Breaded Veal
    Chops
  Baked Sweet Potatoes
  Succotash
  Baking Powder
    Biscuits, hot
  Butter or Margarine—
    Raspberry Jam
  Cabbage and Pineapple
    Salad
  Apple Brown Betty

  Beverage(s)

SUPPER
  Spaghetti with
    Tomato and Meat
    Sauce
  Carrots, glazed
  Mixed Fruit Salad
  Roll, wholewheat
  Butter or Margarine
  Orange Pie
  Beverage(s)

WEDNESDAY

BREAKFAST
  Chilled Pineapple Juice
  Assorted Cold Cereals
    or
  Oatmeal with Cream
  Hot Rolls
  Butter or Margarine
  Jelly
  Beverage(s)

DINNER
  Baked Spanish Steak

  Boiled Potatoes
  Frenched Green Beans
  Tossed Vegetable
    Salad
  Rolls
  Butter or Margarine
  Refrigerator Pudding
  Beverage(s)

SUPPER
  Chicken Soup
  Beef Stroganoff,
    Buttered Noodles

  Stuffed Celery Sticks
  Buttered Peas
  Bread, white or dark
  Butter or Margarine
  Raisin Nut Pudding
  Beverage(s)

THURSDAY	FRIDAY

BREAKFAST
Grapefruit Sections,
　Grenadine
Poached Egg on
　Buttered Toast
Apple Danish Roll
Butter or Margarine
Beverage(s)

BREAKFAST
Chilled Prune Juice
Old Fashioned Waffles
Honey Butter
Warm Maple Syrup
Beverage(s)

DINNER
Broiled Liver
Potatoes au Gratin

Broccoli
Tomato Aspic
　Salad
Rolls
Butter or Margarine
Gingerbread/Whipped
　Cream
Beverage(s)

DINNER
Shrimp Rarebit in
　Cheddar Cheese Sauce
Buttered Carrots and
　Peas
Rolls
Butter or Margarine—
　Jelly
Fresh Strawberry-
　Rhubarb Sauce
Beverage(s)

SUPPER
Cream of Corn
　Soup
Crackers
Assorted Sandwiches
Molded Green Salad

Oatmeal Rocks
　(cookies)
Beverage(s)

SUPPER
Cream of Mushroom
　Soup
Codfish Cakes
French Fries
Stuffed Tomato with
　Apples and Celery
Chilled Apricots
Beverage(s)

SATURDAY

BREAKFAST
> Chilled Fresh Melon
>   Slice
> Assorted Cold Cereals
>   or
> Cream of Wheat,
>   warm milk
> Pecan Roll
> Butter or Margarine
> Beverage(s)

DINNER
> Lamb or Irish Stew
>
> Savory Beets
> Rolls
> Butter or Margarine
> Prune and Carrot Salad
> Bread Pudding with
>   Lemon Sauce
> Beverage(s)

SUPPER
> Potato Onion Soup
> Turkey Cheese Puff
> Malaga Grape and
>   Orange Salad
> Bread, white and dark
> Butter or Margarine
> Date Torte
> Beverage(s)

22nd Week

SUNDAY	MONDAY
BREAKFAST	**BREAKFAST**
Chilled Melon	Assorted Fruit Juices
Scrambled Eggs	Selected Cold Cereals
Hickory Smoked Bacon	or
Cinnamon Raisin Rolls	Oatmeal, with Cream
Beverage(s)	Toast, buttered
	Jelly
	Beverage(s)
DINNER	**DINNER**
Roast Chicken,	Roast Fresh Ham
Dressing	Buttered Parsley Potatoes
Giblet Gravy	Buttered Baby Whole
Mashed Potatoes	Beets
Cauliflower with	Apple Sauce, Warm
Cheese Sauce	Roll
Carrot and Raisin	Butter or Margarine
Salad	Fruit Pudding
Rolls	Custard Sauce
Butter or Margarine	Beverage(s)
Strawberry Shortcake/	
Whipped Cream	
Beverage(s)	
SUPPER	**SUPPER**
Cream of Pea Soup	Cream of Tomato
Assorted Sandwiches	Soup, with
Grapefruit and	croutons
Romaine/Salad	Broiled Veal Pattie
dressing	Marinated Green
Chocolate Pudding	Bean Salad
Beverage(s)	Buttered Broccoli
	Spice Cake, with
	Frosting
	Beverage(s)

TUESDAY

BREAKFAST
 Orange Sections
 Poached Egg on
  Buttered Toast
 Hot Rolls
 Butter or Margarine
 Jam
 Beverage(s)

DINNER
 Barbecued Spareribs

 French Fried
  Potatoes
 Creamed Celery
 Corn Bread—butter
  or margarine
 Cabbage and Green
  Pepper Salad
 Lemon Cream Pie
 Beverage(s)

SUPPER
 Chili Con Carne
 Tossed Crisp Vegetable
  Salad/dressing
 Hard Roll
 Butter or Margarine
 Pineapple Tapioca
 Beverage(s)

WEDNESDAY

BREAKFAST
 Bananas with Cream
 Golden French Toast
 Maple Syrup or Honey
 Canadian Bacon
 Beverage(s)

DINNER
 Salisbury Steak, gravy
 Buttered Parsley Potatoes
 Glazed Carrots
 Wilted Lettuce (bacon
  drippings and vinegar,
  etc.)
 Rolls
 Butter or Margarine
 Chilled Peaches—Cookies
 Beverage(s)

SUPPER
 Cream of Lima
  Bean Soup
 Stuffed Green Pepper
  with Ham and Rice
 Jellied Fruit
  Salad/dressing
 Bread, white and dark
 Butter or Margarine
 Spicy Applesauce Torte
  with Topping
 Beverage(s)

THURSDAY	FRIDAY

BREAKFAST
Assorted Juices
Selected Cold Cereal
    or
Wheatena, with cream
Corn Muffins
Butter or Margarine
Jelly
Beverage(s)

DINNER
Liver Patties
Baked Potato with
    Butter
Fried Parsnips
Buttered Peas
Jellied Vegetable
    Salad Square/
    dressing
Rhubarb Pie
Beverage(s)

SUPPER
Split Pea Soup
Flaky Crusted Beef
    Pot Pie
Peach and Cheese Salad
Parker House Roll
Butter or Margarine
Whipped Orange
    Gelatin/Cream
Beverage(s)

BREAKFAST
Grapefruit Half
Fried Egg
Plantation Sausage
Toast
Butter or Margarine—
    Jam
Beverage(s)

DINNER
Macaroni and
    Cheese
Buttered Peas
Stewed Tomatoes,
    with buttered crumb
    topping
Rolls
Butter or Margarine
Pineapple Upside
    Down Cake/
    Topping
Beverage(s)

SUPPER
Cream of Tomato Soup

Tuna Fish Sandwich
    and
Swiss Cheese Sandwich
Fruit Salad/dressing
Fruited Gelatin
Peanut Butter
Cookies
Beverage(s)

SATURDAY

BREAKFAST
  Assorted Juices
  Buttermilk Pancakes
  Honey Butter
  Warm Maple Syrup
  Canadian Bacon
  Beverage(s)

DINNER
  Ham Loaf with Horse-
    radish Sauce
  Steamed Rice with
    Butter
  Sliced Warm Beets
  Fresh Garden Salad

  Bread, white and dark
  Butter or Margarine
  Baked Apple with
    topping
  Beverage(s)

SUPPER
  French Onion Soup

  Sliced Cold Meat Platter
  Potato Salad
  Buttered Peas and Carrots
  Bread, white and dark
  Butter or Margarine
  Peach Crisp with
    topping
  Beverage(s)

23rd Week

SUNDAY

BREAKFAST
Chilled Orange Juice
Country Fresh Egg
Grilled Sausages
Apple Cinnamon
    Doughnuts
Butter or Margarine
Beverage(s)

DINNER
Fried Chicken
Giblet Gravy
Mashed Potatoes
Baby Lima Beans
Pear/Cream Cheese on
    Lettuce Salad
Corn Meal Rolls
Butter or Margarine
Vanilla Ice Cream/Fresh
    Strawberry Sauce
Beverage(s)

SUPPER
Vegetable Soup
Assorted Cold Meats
    and Cheese
Perfection Salad
    Squares
Potato Chips
Macaroni Salad
Bread, white and dark
Butter or Margarine
Grapenut Custard
Beverage(s)

MONDAY

BREAKFAST
Fruit in Season
Old Fashioned Waffles
Crisp Bacon
Honey or Maple Syrup
Soft Butter
Beverage(s)

DINNER
Braised Beef with
    Potatoes and Carrots

Apple Gelatin Waldorf
    Salad   with
    Lettuce and Dressing
Bran Muffins
Butter or Margarine
Tapioca Pudding with
    Chocolate Sauce
Beverage(s)

SUPPER
Beef Noodle Soup
Turkey Salad with
    Celery and Hard
    Cooked Eggs
Bread, white and dark
Butter or Margarine
Green Beans
Angel Food Cake with
    Butterscotch Sauce

Beverage(s)

TUESDAY	WEDNESDAY
BREAKFAST	**BREAKFAST**

BREAKFAST
Assorted Juices
Poached Egg on
Buttered Toast
Raspberry Danish Roll
Butter or Margarine
Jelly
Beverage(s)

DINNER
Meat Stew with
Dumplings

Buttered Broccoli
Tomato Aspic
Boysenberry Pie
Beverage(s)

SUPPER
Minestrone Soup

Saltines
Italian Spaghetti
with Meat
Sauce
Tossed Green Salad/
French Dressing

French Bread—butter
or margarine
Cinnamon Apple Cup-
cakes/Lemon Sauce
Beverage(s)

BREAKFAST
Half Grapefruit
Selected Cold Cereal
or
Cream of Wheat,
with cream
Golden Toast
Butter or Margarine
Jelly
Beverage(s)

DINNER
Fried Liver and
Bacon
Buttered Parsley
Potatoes
Honey Glazed Carrots
Chef's Salad
Muffins
Butter or Margarine
Coconut Cream Pie
Beverage(s)

SUPPER
Cream of Fresh Carrot
Soup
½ Ham Salad Sandwich
on Rye Bread
½ Egg Salad Sandwich
on Whole Wheat
Bread
Buttered Celery
with Peas
Grapefruit Salad
Graham Cracker
Chocolate Cookies
Beverage(s)

THURSDAY	FRIDAY
BREAKFAST	**BREAKFAST**
Chilled Fruit Juice	Orange Slices
Buttermilk Pancakes	Scrambled Eggs
Soft Butter	Crisp Bacon
Warm Maple Syrup	Toast
or Honey	Butter or Margarine—
Beverage(s)	Jelly
	Beverage(s)

DINNER	**DINNER**
Meat Loaf, gravy	Salmon and Potato
Baked Potatoes and	Casserole, uce
Butter	Parsley Sauce
Corn, creamed style	Brussels Sprouts
Pineapple Cottage	Perfection Salad
Cheese Salad	with
	mayonnaise
Lemon Oatmeal Drop	Rolls
Cookies	Butter or Margarine
Beverage(s)	Bread Pudding with
	Dates and Vanilla
	Sauce
	Beverage(s)

SUPPER	**SUPPER**
V-8 Juice	Cream of Mushroom
Crabmeat Casserole	Soup
Tossed Green Salad	Tomato Stuffed with
	Egg Salad
Bread, white and dark	Potato Chips
Butter or Margarine	Celery and Carrot
Refrigerator Pudding	Curls
Beverage(s)	Bread, white and dark
	Butter or Margarine
	Apple Pie
	Beverage(s)

SATURDAY

BREAKFAST
  Stewed Prunes, Lemon
    Slices
  Assorted Cold Cereals
        or
  Oatmeal, with Cream
  Cinnamon Streusel
    Danish
  Butter or Margarine
  Beverage(s)

DINNER
  Italian Spaghetti and
    Meat Sauce
  Tossed Green Salad/
    dressing
  Poppy Seed Hard Rolls

  Garlic Butter
  Lemon Meringue Pie
  Beverage(s)

SUPPER
  Beef Broth
  Skinned Bologna, Holland
  German Potato Salad,
    hot
  Horseradish-Mustard and
    Catsup
  Green Beans
  Chilled Pears
  Beverage(s)

24th Week

SUNDAY

BREAKFAST
Grapefruit and
   Orange Sections
Bacon Omelet
Golden Toast
Butter or Margarine
Jam or Marmalade
Beverage(s)

DINNER
Roast Loin of
   Pork
Baked Apple Rings
Mashed Sweet Potatoes
Steamed Spinach
Jellied Fruit Salad

Roll
Butter or Margarine
Lemon Sherbet—
   Cookies
Beverage(s)

SUPPER
Chicken Rice Soup
   with Crackers

Cottage Cheese and
   Peach Salad
Raisin Toast
Butter or Margarine
Devils Food Cake,
   Frosted
Beverage(s)

MONDAY

BREAKFAST
Chilled Fruit Juice
Assorted Cold Cereals
   or
Wheatena, with Cream
Cheese Danish Roll
Butter or Margarine
Beverage(s)

DINNER
Baked Beef Hash
   (includes potatoes)

Buttered Green Beans
Creamed Onions
Grapefruit Salad/
   dressing
Rolls
Butter or Margarine
Vanilla Pudding with
   Chocolate Sauce
Beverage(s)

SUPPER
Cream of Celery
   Soup
Tomato, Beef and
   Cheese Sandwiches
Tossed Vegetable
   Salad
Chilled Pear Halves
Beverage(s)

TUESDAY

BREAKFAST
  Stewed Apricots
  Fried Egg
  Hickory Smoked
    Bacon
  Golden Toast
  Butter or Margarine
  Jam
  Beverage(s)

DINNER
  Barbecued Spare Ribs

  Browned Potatoes
  Brussel Sprouts
  French Endive Salad/
    dressing
  Orange Sherbet—
    Cookies
  Beverage(s)

SUPPER
  Creamed Chipped
    Beef on Toast
  Buttered Asparagus
  Jellied Fruit Salad
  Raisin Cookies
  Beverage(s)

WEDNESDAY

BREAKFAST
  Chilled Pineapple Juice
  Assorted Cold Cereals
    or
  Oatmeal, with Cream
  Hot Rolls
  Butter or Margarine
  Jelly
  Beverage(s)

DINNER
  Pan Fried Lamb
    Patties
  Lyonnaise
    Potatoes
  Buttered Peas
  Rolls—Mint Jelly
  Butter or Margarine
  Lettuce and Tomato
    Salad
  Custard Pie
  Beverage(s)

SUPPER
  Corn Chowder
  Cold Meat Salad
    Sandwich
  Baked Lima Beans
    in Tomato Sauce
  Perfection Salad
    Squares
  Baked Rice Pudding
    with Apricot Sauce
  Beverage(s)

THURSDAY	FRIDAY

THURSDAY

BREAKFAST
   Grapefruit Sections,
     Grenadine
   Poached Egg on
     Buttered Toast
   Apple Danish Roll
   Butter or Margarine
   Beverage(s)

DINNER
   Chicken Fricassee
   Dumplings and Gravy

   French Green Beans,
     Buttered
   Jellied Fruit Salad

   Red Raspberry Sherbet—
     Cookies
   Beverage(s)

SUPPER
   Bouillon
   Fried Sausage Links
   Baked Potato
   Mixed Vegetables
   Bread—Butter or
     Margarine
   Yellow Cupcakes
     with Icing
   Beverage(s)

FRIDAY

BREAKFAST
   Chilled Prune Juice
   Old Fashioned Waffles
   Honey Butter
   Warm Maple Syrup
   Beverage(s)

DINNER
   Salmon Loaf Florentine
   Whipped Potatoes
   Buttered Mixed
     Vegetables
   Stuffed Celery Sticks

   Bread, white and dark
   Butter or Margarine
   Nut and Raisin
     Cookies
   Beverage(s)

SUPPER
   Cream of Asparagus
     Soup
   Assorted Sandwiches
   Buttered, Whole Kernel
     Corn
   Grated Carrot and
     Raisin Salad
   Chocolate Pudding
   Beverage(s)

SATURDAY

BREAKFAST
  Chilled Fresh Melon
    Slice
  Assorted Cold Cereals
    or
  Cream of Wheat,
    warm milk
  Cinnamon Raisin
    Pecan Roll
  Butter or Margarine
  Beverage(s)

DINNER
  Corned Beef and
    Cabbage
  Boiled Potatoes
  Molded Vegetable
    Salad
  Rye Bread
  Butter or Margarine
  Baked Custard
  Beverage(s)

SUPPER
  Vegetable Soup
  Bologna Sandwich on
    Black Bread—White
    Bread
  Butter or Margarine
  Hot German Potato
    Salad
  Mustard—Catsup
  Brown Sugar Cake
  Beverage(s)

25th Week

SUNDAY	MONDAY
BREAKFAST	**BREAKFAST**
Chilled Melon	Assorted Fruit Juices
Scrambled Eggs	Selected Cold Cereals
Hickory Smoked	or
Bacon	Oatmeal, with Cream
Honey Dip Dough-	Toast, buttered
nuts	Jelly
Beverage(s)	Beverage(s)
DINNER	**DINNER**
Tomato Juice	Meat Balls in
Roast Beef	Mushroom Sauce
Oven Browned	
Potatoes	Hashed Brown Potatoes
Beets with Orange	
Sauce	Parslied Cole Slaw
Cabbage, Apple and	Carrots, shoestring
Pineapple Salad	style
	Bread, white and dark
Cloverleaf Rolls	Butter or Margarine
Butter or Margarine	Fluffy White Cake,
Gelatin with Mixed	Orange Cream
Fruit, Whipped	Frosting
Topping	Beverage(s)
Beverage(s)	
SUPPER	**SUPPER**
Cream of Mushrrom	Chicken Rice
Soup	Soup
Hamburger on Bun	Beef Stew
Celery Sticks	on Hot Biscuit
Pickles—Relish	Apple and Celery Salad
Strawberry Short-	Bran Applesauce
cake	Cookies
Beverage(s)	Beverage(s)

TUESDAY	WEDNESDAY

BREAKFAST
- Orange Sections
- Poached Egg on
  - Buttered Toast
- Hot Rolls
- Butter or Margarine
- Jam
- Beverage(s)

DINNER
- Baked Stuffed
  - Pork Chop
- Whipped Potatoes
- Buttered Spinach
- Corn Muffins,
  - Apple Jelly
- Butter or Margarine
- Whipped Fruit
  - Gelatin
- Beverage(s)

SUPPER
- Beef Noodle Soup
- Chicken Salad
- Bread, white and dark
- Potato Chips
- Tossed Vegetable Salad/
  - Russian Dressing
- Butter or Margarine
- Dutch Apple Cake
- Beverage(s)

BREAKFAST
- Bananas with Cream
- Golden French Toast
- Maple Syrup or Honey
- Canadian Bacon
- Beverage(s)

DINNER
- Pot Roast of Beef

- Cottage Fried Potatoes
- Diced Summer Squash
  - in Sour Cream
- Fresh Green Beans
- Cucumber Slices/
  - Vinegar and Oil
- Apple Betty
- Beverage(s)

SUPPER
- French Onion
  - Soup
- Braised Liver and
  - Bacon
- Asparagus, creamed
- Bread, white and dark
- Butter or Margarine
- Old Fashioned Rice
  - Pudding
- Beverage(s)

THURSDAY	FRIDAY

BREAKFAST
- Assorted Juices
- Selected Cold Cereal
  - or
- Wheatena, with Cream
- Blueberry Muffin
- Butter or Margarine
  - Jelly
- Beverage(s)

BREAKFAST
- Grapefruit Half
- Fried Egg
- Plantation Sausage
- Toast
- Butter or Margarine
- Jam
- Beverage(s)

DINNER
- Salisbury Steak
- Buttered Noodles
- Harvard Beets
- Carrot and Raisin
  - Salad
- Rolls
- Butter or Margarine
- Peach Cobbler
- Beverage(s)

DINNER
- Fried Filet of Perch
- Au Gratin
  - Potatoes
- Buttered Green Peas
- Tomato Aspic
- Rolls
- Butter or Margarine
- Lemon Meringue Pie
- Beverage(s)

SUPPER
- Minestrone Soup

- Spaghetti with
  - Tomato-Meat
  - Sauce
- Tossed Green Salad/
  - Italian Dressing
- French Bread
- Butter or Margarine
- Chilled Pears
- Beverage(s)

SUPPER
- Vegetable Soup
- Tunafish Salad
  - Sandwiches
- Potato Chips
- Mixed Green Salad/
  - French Dressing
- Pineapple Cheese Cake

- Beverage(s)

SATURDAY

BREAKFAST
  Assorted Juices
  Buttermilk Pancakes
  Honey Butter
  Warm Maple Syrup
  Grilled Ham
  Beverage(s)

DINNER
  Braised Short Ribs of
      Beef with natural
      gravy
  Mashed Potatoes
  Buttered String Beans
  Lettuce Salad/Thousand
      Isalnd Dressing
  Bread, white and dark
  Butter or Margarine
  Creamed Coconut Cake
  Beverage(s)

SUPPER
  Tomato Soup
  Escalloped Ham and
      Potatoes
  Lima Beans
  Jellied Fruit Salad
  Rolls
  Butter or Margarine
  Refrigerator Pudding
  Beverage(s)

26th Week

SUNDAY	MONDAY

BREAKFAST
Chilled Orange Juice
Country Fresh Egg
Grilled Sausages
Almond Nut
Doughnuts
Butter or Margarine
Beverage(s)

DINNER
Baked Virginia
Ham
Baked Yams with
Butter
Peas, Buttered
Tossed Salad/
dressing
Rolls
Butter or Margarine
Peach Shortcake/
Topping
Beverage(s)

SUPPER
Vegetable Soup
Pizza
Buttered Green
Beans, french style
Pineapple Sherbet
Beverage(s)

BREAKFAST
Fruit in Season
Old Fashioned Waffles
Crisp Bacon
Honey or Maple Syrup
Soft Butter
Beverage(s)

DINNER
Beef Pot Roast
Buttered Noodles
Glazed Carrot
Rings
Cheese Biscuits—Butter
or Margarine
Cabbage and Apple
Salad
Butterscotch Pudding
Beverage(s)

SUPPER
Spanish Rice and Bacon
Peach-Cottage Cheese
Salad
Bread, white and dark
Butter or Margarine
Nut and Raisin
Cookies
Beverage(s)

TUESDAY

BREAKFAST
　Assorted Juices
　Poached Egg on
　　Buttered Toast
　Orange Danish Roll
　Butter or Margarine
　Jelly
　Beverage(s)

DINNER
　Breaded Veal Cutlet
　　　with Tomato
　　Sauce
　Mashed Potatoes
　Vegetable Medley
　　Salad
　Carrots and Peas
　Rolls
　Butter or Margarine
　Butterscotch Pie
　Beverage(s)

SUPPER
　Sweet and Sour Pork
　Buttered Rice
　Green Tossed Salad/
　　dressing
　Roll, wholewheat
　Butter or Margarine
　Whipped Gelatin
　　with Bananas
　Beverage(s)

WEDNESDAY

BREAKFAST
　Half Grapefruit
　Selected Cold Cereal
　　or
　Cream of Wheat,
　　with cream
　Golden Toast
　Butter or Margarine–
　　Jelly
　Beverage(s)

DINNER
　Swiss Steak
　Buttered Noodles
　Spinach
　Lettuce and
　　Tomato Salad
　Rolls
　Butter or Margarine
　Chocolate
　　Brownies
　Beverage(s)

SUPPER
　Cream of Celery
　　Soup
　Meat Salad Plate
　Chef's Salad, French
　　Dressing
　Potato Chips
　Bread, white and dark
　Butter or Margarine
　Apricot Whip
　Beverage(s)

THURSDAY	FRIDAY

BREAKFAST
Chilled Fruit Juice
Buttermilk Pancakes
Soft Butter
Warm Maple Syrup
  or Honey
Beverage(s)

BREAKFAST
Orange Slices
Scrambled Eggs
Crisp Bacon
Toast
Butter or Margarine—
  Jelly
Beverage(s)

DINNER
Braised Beef and
  Vegetables
Baked Potato
Perfection Salad
Bread, white and dark
Butter or Margarine
Baked Custard
Beverage(s)

DINNER
Baked Fillet of
  Fish   with
  Spanish Sauce
French Fried Potatoes
Green Beans, french
  style
Molded Beet Salad
Bread, white and dark
Butter or Margarine
Chocolate Chip
  Cookies
Beverage(s)

SUPPER
Grilled Frankfurter
  on Bun
German Potato
  Salad
Relishes and Pickles
Three Bean Salad
Ice Cream—Cookies
Beverage(s)

SUPPER
Cream of Mushroom
  Soup
Assorted Sandwiches
Summer Fruit Salad/
  dressing
Coconut Pudding
Beverage(s)

SATURDAY

BREAKFAST
  Stewed Prunes,
     Lemon Slices
  Assorted Cold Cereals
        or
  Oatmeal, with Cream
  Cherry Streusel Danish
  Butter or Margarine
  Beverage(s)

DINNER
  Corned Beef and
     Cabbage
  Boiled Potatoes
  Cottage Cheese Salad
  Rolls
  Butter or Margarine
  Applesauce Cake/
     Topping
  Beverage(s)

SUPPER
  Beef Broth
  Chef's Salad Bowl
  Pickles—Olives—Radishes
  Jellied Fruit Salad
  Toffee Squares (cookies)
  Beverage(s)

27th Week

SUNDAY	MONDAY
BREAKFAST	**BREAKFAST**
Grapefruit and	Chilled Fruit Juice
Orange Sections	Assorted Cold Cereals
Bacon Omelet	or
Golden Toast	Wheatena, with Cream
Butter or Margarine	Cheese Danish Roll
Jam or Marmalade	Butter or Margarine
Beverage(s)	Beverage(s)
DINNER	**DINNER**
Roast Loin of	V-8 Juice
Pork	Veal Pot Pie, flaky crust
Mashed Potatoes	Mashed Potatoes
Broccoli Spears,	Creamed Spinach
buttered	Bread, white and dark
Warm Applesauce	Butter or Margarine
Rolls	Pineapple Cake
Butter or Margarine	Beverage(s)
Ice Cream—Cookies	
Beverage(s)	
SUPPER	**SUPPER**
Corned Beef Hash	Cream of Mushroom
with Poached Egg	Soup
Gingerale Fruit Salad/	Baked Omelet with
dressing	Currant Jelly
Roll, wholewheat	Jellied Fruit Salad
Butter or Margarine	Bread, white and dark
Yellow Pound Cake	Butter or Margarine
Beverage(s)	Chocolate Fudge
	Cookies
	Beverage(s)

TUESDAY

BREAKFAST
Stewed Apricots
Fried Egg
Hickory Smoked
Bacon
Golden Toast
Butter or Margarine—
Jam
Beverage(s)

DINNER
Liver and Bacon
French Fried Onion
Rings
Parsley Buttered
Potatoes
Spiced Peach Salad
Bread
Butter or Margarine
Sponge Cake/
Topping
Beverage(s)

SUPPER
Tomato Bouillon
Main Dish—Fruit
Salad with Cottage
Cheese
Raisin Toast
Butter or Margarine
Pineapple Sherbet,
Spice Cookies
Beverage(s)

WEDNESDAY

BREAKFAST
Chilled Pineapple Juice
Assorted Cold Cereals
or
Oatmeal, with Cream
Hot Rolls
Butter or Margarine
Jelly
Beverage(s)

DINNER
Chicken, oven
fried
Baked Potato
Creamed Peas and
Carrots
Wilted Lettuce
Salad/Bacon
dressing
Rolls
Butter or Margarine
Chocolate Fudge
Cake /Icing
Beverage(s)

SUPPER
Navy Bean Soup
Brown Bread and
Cream Cheese
Sandwiches
Jellied Fruit Salad/
dressing
Baked Rice Custard
Beverage(s)

THURSDAY

BREAKFAST
Grapefruit Sections,
  Grenadine
Poached Egg on
  Buttered Toast
Apple Danish Roll
Butter or Margarine
Beverage(s)

DINNER
Spareribs and Sauer-
  kraut
Boiled Potatoes
Buttered Carrots
Jellied Fruit Salad
Wholewheat Bread
Butter or Margarine
Chilled Pears
Beverage(s)

SUPPER
Split Pea Soup
  and Crackers
Potato Pancakes
Mixed Vegetable
  Garden Salad/
  dressing
Peach Halves, chilled
Vanilla Cookies
Beverage(s)

FRIDAY

BREAKFAST
Chilled Prune Juice
Old Fashioned Waffles
Honey Butter
Warm Maple Syrup
Beverage(s)

DINNER
Creamed Tunafish over
  Buttered Baking
  Powder Biscuit
Green Beans with
  Pimiento Strips
Summer Green Salad/
  dressing
Butterscotch Pudding
Beverage(s)

SUPPER
Manhattan Clam
  Chowder
Toasted Cheese Sand-
  wich
Buttered Green Peas
Jellied Fruit Salad
Cream Puff
Beverage(s)

SATURDAY

BREAKFAST
    Chilled Fresh Melon
       Slice
    Assorted Cold Cereals
       or
    Cream of Wheat,
       warm milk
    Cinnamon Raisin Pecan
       Roll
    Butter or Margarine
    Beverage(s)

DINNER
    Italian Spaghetti with
       Meat Sauce
    Tossed Green Salad
    Hard Rolls, poppy seed

    Butter or Margarine
    Baked Cherry Pudding/
       Topping
    Beverage(s)

SUPPER
    Beef Broth and
       Crackers
    Chicken Salad Sandwiches
    Potato Chips
    Assorted Pickles and
       Relishes
    Coconut Custard Cup
    Beverage(s)

28th Week

SUNDAY	MONDAY
BREAKFAST	**BREAKFAST**
Chilled Melon	Assorted Fruit
Scrambled Eggs	Selected Cold Cereals
Hickory Smoked	or
Bacon	Oatmeal, with Cream
Cinnamon Toast	Raised Doughnut
Butter or Margarine	Beverage(s)
Beverage(s)	
DINNER	**DINNER**
Roast Turkey	Meat Loaf, gravy
stuffing	Fried Potatoes
Giblet Gravy	Spiced Hot Beets
Mashed Potatoes	Escalloped Onions
Parsnips, browned	Rolls
Peas	Butter or Margarine
Waldorf Salad	Chilled Melon
Raisin Bread	Beverage(s)
Butter or Margarine	
Strawberry Pie	
Beverage(s)	
SUPPER	**SUPPER**
Cream of Asparagus	Potato Soup with
Soup	Chives
Turkey Salad	Sliced Corned Beef
Assorted Relishes—	Sandwiches
Pickles—Olives	Pickles—Relishes—
Potato Chips	Cole Slaw
Bread, raisin and whole-	Applesauce
wheat	Beverage(s)
Butter or Margarine	
Whipped Fruit Gelatin	
Beverage(s)	

TUESDAY

BREAKFAST
    Orange Sections
    Poached Egg on
        Buttered Toast
    Hot Rolls
    Butter or Margarine
    Jam
    Beverage(s)

DINNER
    Veal Stew
    Hard Crusty Rolls
    Butter or Margarine—
        Jelly
    Cabbage and Pineapple
        Salad
    Orange Ice
    Beverage(s)

SUPPER
Barley Tomato Soup
Assorted Cold Meats
    and Cheese
Potato Salad
Succotash
Bread, white and dark
Butter or Margarine
Jelly Roll
Beverage(s)

WEDNESDAY

BREAKFAST
    Bananas with Cream
    Golden French Toast
    Maple Syrup or Honey
    Canadian Bacon
    Beverage(s)

DINNER
    Fricassee of Lamb,
        Buttered Rice
    Corn Bread
    Butter or Margarine
    Spiced Beets
    Prune and Carrot
        Salad
    Chilled Apricots
    Beverage(s)

SUPPER
    Chicken and Rice
        Soup
    Frankfurters on Hot
        Rolls
    French Fried Potatoes
    Relishes—Catsup
    Apple and Celery
        Salad
    Fluffy White Cake
        with Chocolate
        Frosting
    Beverage(s)

THURSDAY

BREAKFAST
Assorted Juices
Selected Cold Cereal
or
Wheatena, with Cream
Corn Muffins
Butter or Margarine
Jelly
Beverage(s)

DINNER
Cubed Liver with
Onion Gravy
Potatoes au Gratin
Broccoli with Lemon
Butter
Jellied Apple and Grape
Salad
Bread, white and dark
Butter or Margarine
Coconut Cream Pudding
Beverage(s)

SUPPER
Cream of Corn Soup
Grilled Hamburger
on Bun, with slice
of onion served
separately
Catsup
Baked Tomato
Butter or Margarine
Apple Crisp
Beverage(s)

FRIDAY

BREAKFAST
Grapefruit Half
Fried Egg
Plantation Sausage
Toast
Butter or Margarine
Jam
Beverage(s)

DINNER
Fried Scallops
with Tartar
Sauce
Baked Potato
Fresh Spinach with
Hard Cooked Egg
Garnish
Tomato and Lettuce
Salad/dressing
Lime Snow
Beverage(s)

SUPPER
Fisherman's Soup
Tunafish Salad
Potato Chips
Cabbage-Apple-Pine-
apple Salad
Olives—Pickles
Banana Cream Pie
Beverage(s)

SATURDAY

BREAKFAST
Assorted Juices
Buttermilk Pancakes
Honey Butter
Warm Maple Syrup
Grilled Ham
Beverage(s)

DINNER
V-8 Juice
Baked Manicotti
Buttered Green Beans
Bread, white and dark
Butter or Margarine
Tossed Green Salad/
    dressing
Chilled Watermelon
Beverage(s)

SUPPER
Cream of Peanut Butter
    Soup
Cheese Sandwich on
   Whole Wheat Bread
Shredded Lettuce with
    dressing
Apple Turnover
Beverage(s)

29th Week

SUNDAY	MONDAY

BREAKFAST
Chilled Orange Juice
Country Fresh Egg
Grilled Sausages
Honey Dip Dough-
nuts
Beverage(s)

BREAKFAST
Fruit in Season
Old Fashioned Waffles
Crisp Bacon
Honey or Maple Syrup
Soft Butter
Beverage(s)

DINNER
Pork Loin Roast,
gravy
Baked Sweet Potato
Tomato and Celery
Sauce
Spiced Apple Rings
Banana and Ground
Nut Salad/dressing

Rolls
Butter or Margarine
Lemon Sherbet
Beverage(s)

DINNER
Veal Parmigiana
Baked Potato
Buttered Brussel
Sprouts
Rolls
Butter or Margarine
Green Salad/dressing

Cherry Pudding
Beverage(s)

SUPPER
Cream of Mushroom
Soup
Ham and Cheese Sand-
wich on whole
wheat bread
Tossed Green Salad/
dressing
Custard Pie
Beverage(s)

SUPPER
Beef Soup with Rice
Baked Hash
Marinated Bean Salad
Bread, white and dark
Butter or Margarine
Mixed Fruit, Upside
Down Cake
Beverage(s)

TUESDAY	**WEDNESDAY**

BREAKFAST
Assorted Juices
Poached Egg on
Buttered Toast
Orange Pineapple Danish
Roll
Butter or Margarine
Beverage(s)

BREAKFAST
Half Grapefruit
Selected Cold Cereals
or
Cream of Wheat,
with cream
Golden Toast
Butter or Margarine
Jelly
Beverage(s)

DINNER
Hungarian Goulash
Buttered Noodles
Julienne Green Beans
Black Bread
Butter or Margarine
Sections of Orange and
Grapefruit on Lettuce/
dressing (230)
Chocolate Cake
Beverage(s)

DINNER
Hamburger Steak
Fried Potatoes
Creamed Onions
with Pimiento
Summer Squash
Rolls
Butter or Margarine
Chilled Peaches
Beverage(s)

SUPPER
Pineapple Juice
Creamed Egg and
Crumbled Bacon
on Toast
Tossed Green Salad

Lemon Refrigerator
Dessert
Beverage(s)

SUPPER
Vegetable Soup
Meat Croquettes
with Horseradish
Sauce
Buttered Chopped
Spinach
Bread, white and dark
Butter or Margarine
Cup Custard
Beverage(s)

THURSDAY	FRIDAY

BREAKFAST
- Chilled Fruit Juice
- Buttermilk Pancakes
- Soft Butter
- Warm Maple Syrup
  - or Honey
- Beverage(s)

DINNER
- Baked Thuringer
  - Sausage with
  - Sauerkraut
- Boiled Potatoes
- Lima Beans
- Tomato and Lettuce
  - Salad/dressing
- Bread, wholewheat
- Butter or Margarine
- Orange and Grapefruit
  - Sections
- Beverage(s)

SUPPER
- Potato and Leek
  - Soup
- Ham Salad Sandwiches
- Jellied Fruit Salad/
  - dressing
- Orange Squares
- Beverage(s)

BREAKFAST
- Orange Slices
- Scrambled Eggs
- Crisp Bacon
- Toast
- Butter or Margarine
- Jelly
- Beverage(s)

DINNER
- Oven Fried Fish
  - Patties,
  - Tartar Sauce
- Buttered Parsley
  - Potatoes
- Fresh Carrots
- Cole Slaw
- Rolls
- Butter or Margarine
- Hot Bread Pudding
  - with Raisins and
  - Vanilla Sauce
- Beverage(s)

SUPPER
- Clam Chowder
- Macaroni and Cheese
  - Loaf   with
  - Tomato Sauce
- Stuffed Celery
- Rolls, wholewheat
- Butter or Margarine
- Fruit Bavarian
- Beverage(s)

SATURDAY

BREAKFAST
Stewed Prunes,
Lemon Slices
Assorted Cold Cereals
or
Oatmeal, with cream
Jelly Doughnuts
Beverage(s)

DINNER
American Chop Suey
with Steamed Rice
Baked Squash, (use
brown sugar)
Pickled Sliced Beets
Rolls
Butter or Margarine
Date Bar
Beverage(s)

SUPPER
Scotch Broth with
Barley and Crackers

Hamburger Pie with
Potato Fluff
Bread
Butter or Margarine
Fruited Gelatin /
topping
Beverage(s)

30th Week

SUNDAY

BREAKFAST
Grapefruit and
Orange Sections
Bacon Omelet
Golden Toast
Butter or Margarine
Jam or Marmalade
Beverage(s)

DINNER
Roast Beef, Gravy
Boiled Potatoes
Scalloped Corn
Buttered Small Beets
Roll
Butter or Margarine
Strawberry Shortcake/
Topping
Beverage(s)

SUPPER
Turkey Noodle Soup
Assorted Cold Sand-
wiches
Catsup and Mustard
Pickles and Olives
Raw Carrot and
Raisin Salad
Peach Custard
Beverage(s)

MONDAY

BREAKFAST
Chilled Fruit Juice
Assorted Cold Cereals
or
Wheatena, with cream
Apricot Danish Roll
Butter or Margarine
Beverage(s)

DINNER
Barbecued Pork Chops
Baked Rice
Buttered Green Peas
Tossed Green Salad/
dressing
Corn Muffins
Butter or Margarine
Whipped Fruit Gelatin
Beverage(s)

SUPPER
Cream of Asparagus
Soup
Deviled Egg Sand-
wiches
Cole Slaw
Olives
Jam Crunchies
Beverage(s)

TUESDAY

BREAKFAST
  Stewed Apricots
  Fried Egg
  Hickory Smoked
    Bacon
  Golden Toast
  Butter or Margarine
  Jam
  Beverage(s)

DINNER
  Roast Turkey
    Stuffing
  Giblet Gravy
  Mashed Potatoes
  Julienne String Beans
  Cranberry Sauce
  Cherrynut Bread
  Butter or Margarine
  Chilled Pear Halves
  Beverage(s)

SUPPER
  Vegetable Soup
  Ham Salad Sandwich
    on wholewheat bread
  Glazed Carrots
  Jellied Waldorf Salad
    (Apple gelatin)
  Peanut Butter
    Cookies
  Beverage(s)

WEDNESDAY

BREAKFAST
  Chilled Pineapple Juice
  Assorted Cold Cereals
    or
  Oatmeal, with cream
  Hot Rolls
  Butter or Margarine—
    Jelly
  Beverage(s)

DINNER
  Braised Calves
    Liver
  Parsley Buttered
    Potatoes
  Stewed Tomato with
    Bread Crumb
    Topping
  Spiced Peach Salad
  Rolls
  Butter or Margarine
  Yellow Sponge Cake

  Beverage(s)

SUPPER
  Cream of Chicken
    Soup
  Tamale Pie
  Spinach
  Jellied Bing
    Cherry Salad
  Blueberry Tarts
  Beverage(s)

THURSDAY	FRIDAY

BREAKFAST
Grapefruit Sections,
   Grenadine
Poached Egg on
   Buttered Toast
Apple Danish Roll
Butter or Margarine
Beverage(s)

BREAKFAST
Chilled Prune Juice
Old Fashioned Waffles
Honey Butter
Warm Maple Syrup
Beverage(s)

DINNER
Veal Roast
Buttered Rice
Creamed Spinach
Tomato Aspic
Rolls
Butter or Margarine
Pineapple-Graham
   Cracker Refrigerator
   Pudding
Beverage(s)

DINNER
Baked Fish Fillet
Buttered Parsley
   Potatoes
Creamed Spinach
Molded Carrot and
   Pineapple Salad
Corn Muffins
Butter or Margarine–
   Apple Butter
Chilled Queen Anne
   Cherries
Beverage(s)

SUPPER
Beef Bouillon
Stuffed Green Peppers
Buttered Brussel
   Sprouts
Bread, white and dark
Butter or Margarine
Chilled Peaches
Beverage(s)

SUPPER
Cream of Tomato
   Soup
Macaroni and Cheese
   Casserole
Buttered Green Beans
Shredded Cabbage
   Salad
Roll
Butter or Margarine
Gingerbread with
   Lemon Sauce
Beverage(s)

SATURDAY

BREAKFAST
Chilled Fresh Melon
Slice
Assorted Cold Cereals
or
Cream of Wheat,
warm milk
Cinnamon Raisin
Pecan Roll
Butter or Margarine
Beverage(s)

DINNER
Roast Lamb
Shoulder
Candied Sweet
Potatoes
Buttered Broccoli
Mixed Vegetable Salad

Poppy Seed Roll
(small)
Butter or Margarine
Norwegian Prune Pudding
Beverage(s)

SUPPER
Spanish Rice with Meat
Frenched Green Beans
Bread, white and dark
Butter or Margarine
Banana Cake with
Icing
Beverage(s)

31st Week

SUNDAY

BREAKFAST
Chilled Melon
Scrambled Eggs
Hickory Smoked
    Bacon
Strawberry Filled
    Doughnuts
Beverage(s)

DINNER
Virginian Baked
    Chicken
Mashed Potatoes and
    Gravy
Jellied Cranberry and
    Orange Salad
June Peas
Rolls
Butter or Margarine
Raspberry Sherbet—
    Cookies
Beverage(s)

SUPPER
Vegetable Soup
Assorted Sandwiches
Sauteed New Carrots
Peach Shortcake
Beverage(s)

MONDAY

BREAKFAST
Assorted Fruit Juices
Selected Cold Cereals
    or
Oatmeal, with cream
Toast, Buttered
Jelly
Beverage(s)

DINNER
Barbecued Beef Hash
    (potatoes included)
Creamed Celery
Buttered Spinach
Bread, white and dark
Butter or Margarine
Angel Food Cake—
    Icing
Beverage(s)

SUPPER
Split Pea Soup
Cold Cuts of Meat
    and Deviled Eggs
Garden Salad/
    dressing
Bread, white and dark
Butter or Margarine
Chilled Pineapple
Beverage(s)

TUESDAY

BREAKFAST
Orange Sections
Poached Egg on
   Buttered Toast
Hot Rolls
Butter or Margarine—
   Jam
Beverage(s)

DINNER
Veal Shoulder,
   Bread Stuffing
Gravy
Mashed Potatoes
Carrot and Raisin
   Salad
Buttered Cauliflower
Rolls
Butter or Margarine
Blueberry Pie
Beverage(s)

SUPPER
Apple Cider
Grilled Cheese
   Sandwich
Carrot and Pineapple
   Salad
Olives and Pickles
Peach Pudding
Cookies
Beverage(s)

WEDNESDAY

BREAKFAST
Bananas with Cream
Golden French Toast
Maple Syrup or Honey
Canadian Bacon
Beverage(s)

DINNER
Leg of Lamb, brown
   gravy
Mint Jelly
Escalloped Potatoes

Buttered Green Beans,
   French Style
Sliced Pineapple and
   Grated Cheese Salad
Bread, white and dark
Butter or Margarine
Vanilla Cookies
Beverage(s)

SUPPER
Beef Noodle Soup
Bacon, Tomato and
   Lettuce Sandwich
   on Toast
Fresh Summer Fruit
   Salad
Custard Pie
   Beverage(s)

THURSDAY

BREAKFAST
　　Assorted Juices
　　Selected Cold Cereal
　　　　or
　　Wheatena, with cream
　　Corn Muffins
　　Butter or Margarine
　　Jelly
　　Beverage(s)

DINNER
　　Braised Short Ribs
　　　with Buttered
　　　Noodles
　　Southern Zucchini
　　　Squash
　　Snap Green Beans
　　Rolls
　　Butter or Margarine
　　Cherry Pie
　　Beverage(s)

SUPPER
　　Cream of Potato
　　　Soup
　　Roast Frankfurters
　　　(stuffed with cheese
　　　and wrapped in bacon)
　　Chilled Cole Slaw
　　Hot Weiner Buns
　　Butter or Margarine
　　Corn Syrup Brownies
　　Beverage(s)

FRIDAY

BREAKFAST
　　Grapefruit Half
　　Fried Egg
　　Plantation Sausage
　　Toast
　　Butter or Margarine—
　　　Jam
　　Beverage(s)

DINNER
　　Breaded Fish Fillets

　　Tartar Sauce
　　Oven Browned
　　　Potatoes
　　Cole Slaw
　　Green Beans,
　　　French Style
　　Rolls, graham
　　Butter or Margarine
　　Apple Souffle
　　Beverage(s)

SUPPER
　　Cream of Asparagus
　　　Soup
　　Peach and Cottage
　　　Cheese Salad
　　　(main dish)
　　Toasted Raisin Bread
　　Strawberry Shortcake

　　Beverage(s)

SATURDAY

BREAKFAST
  Assorted Juices
  Buttermilk Pancakes
  Honey Butter
  Warm Maple Syrup
  Grilled Ham
  Beverage(s)

DINNER
  Baked Shoulder
    Lamb Chops
  Parsley Potatoes
  Tomato and Celery Sauce
  Tossed Green Salad/
    dressing
  Rolls
  Butter or Margarine
  Cup Custard
  Beverage(s)

SUPPER
  Cream of Mushroom
    Soup
  Pork Sausage Patties
  Hot Potato Salad
  Bread, white or dark
  Butter or Margarine
  Devils Food Cake
  Beverage(s)

32nd Week

SUNDAY	MONDAY

BREAKFAST
    Chilled Orange Juice
    Country Fresh Egg
    Grilled Sausages
    Almond Nut Dough-
       nuts
    Butter or Margarine
    Beverage(s)

BREAKFAST
    Fruit in Season
    Old Fashioned Waffles
    Crisp Bacon
    Honey or Maple Syrup
    Soft Butter
    Beverage(s)

DINNER
    Southern Fried Chicken
       and Gravy
    Mashed Potatoes
    Buttered Asparagus
    Jellied Fruit Salad
    Hot Rolls
    Butter or Margarine
    Chocolate Cream Pie
    Beverage(s)

DINNER
    Roast Beef, Natural
       Gravy
    Oven Browned
       Potatoes
    Cauliflower, buttered
    Tossed Green Salad

    Bread, white and dark
    Butter or Margarine
    Chilled Pears
    Beverage(s)

SUPPER
    Beef Noodle Soup
    Cold Meat Plate
    Sliced Tomato on
       Watercress/dress-
       ing
    Bread, white and dark
    Butter or Margarine
    Potato Chips
    Vanilla Ice Cream
    Beverage(s)

SUPPER
    Spaghetti with Tomato
       Meat Sauce
    Buttered Lima Beans
    Italian Bread
    Butter or Margarine
    Chocolate Cream Pie
    Beverage(s)

TUESDAY

BREAKFAST
Assorted Juices
Poached Egg on
  Buttered Toast
Orange Pineapple Danish
  Roll
Butter or Margarine,
  Jelly
Beverage(s)

DINNER
Braised Calves Liver
  and Onions
Parsley Buttered
  Potatoes
Breaded Tomatoes
Stuffed Celery
Rolls, graham
Fruit Whip
Beverage(s)

SUPPER
Minestrone Soup
Holland Style
  Bologna
Sour Black Bread
Catsup and Horse-
  radish Mustard
Butter or Margarine
Jellied Pineapple and
  Carrot Salad
Coconut Macaroons
Beverage(s)

WEDNESDAY

BREAKFAST
Half Grapefruit
Selected Cold Cereal
  or
Cream of Wheat,
  with cream
Golden Toast
Butter or Margarine,
  Jelly
Beverage(s)

DINNER
American Chop Suey
  with Chinese Noodles
Buttered Rice
Peas and Carrots
Pink Grapefruit Salad
  on Lettuce/dressing

Rolls
Butter or Margarine
Burnt Almond
  Sponge Cake
Beverage(s)

SUPPER
Vegetable Beef Soup

Chicken Shortcake
Jellied Fruit Salad
Oatmeal Drop
  Cookies
Beverage(s)

THURSDAY	**FRIDAY**

BREAKFAST
Chilled Fruit Juice
Buttermilk Pancakes
Soft Butter
Warm Maple Syrup
   or Honey
Beverage(s)

BREAKFAST
Orange Slices
Scrambled Eggs
Crisp Bacon
Toast
Butter or Margarine—
   Jelly
Beverage(s)

DINNER
Baked Swiss Steak
Baked Potato with
   Butter or Sour
   Cream (Commercial)
Cauliflower Polonaise,
   Parsley Topping
Crisp Green Salad
   Bowl
Cranberries, jellied
Rolls
Butter or Margarine
Peach Melba
Beverage(s)

DINNER
Broiled Halibut
Lemon Wedges
French Fried Potatoes
Glazed Carrot Rings

Coleslaw
Sesame Seed Rolls
Butter or Margarine
Red Cherry Torte
Beverage(s)

SUPPER
Apple Juice
Pork Sausage Patties
Spinach with crumbled
   Bacon Sauce
Tomato Slices on
   Lettuce Leaf/
   dressing
Watermelon
Beverage(s)

SUPPER
Tuna Fish a la King
   on Toast surrounded
   with Peas
Molded Spiced Fruit
   Salad
Chilled Apricots
Peanut Butter
   Cookies
Beverage(s)

SATURDAY

BREAKFAST
 Stewed Prunes,
  Lemon Slices
 Assorted Cold Cereals
  or
 Oatmeal, with Cream
 Blueberry Streusel
  Danish
 Butter or Margarine
 Beverage(s)

DINNER
 Meat Loaf, Gravy
 Scalloped Potatoes
 Buttered Spinach and
  Bacon
 Waldorf Salad
 Rolls, wholewheat
 Butter or Margarine
 Pumpkin Cookies
 Beverage(s)

SUPPER
 Chicken Soup with
  Noodles
 Hot Frankfurter on
  Bun
 Potato Salad
 Buttered Carrots
 Pickles, Mustard,
  Catsup
 Baked Rice Custard
 Beverage(s)

33rd Week

SUNDAY

BREAKFAST
Grapefruit and
Orange Sections
Bacon Omelet
Golden Toast
Butter or Margarine
Jam or Marmalade
Beverage(s)

DINNER
Old Fashioned
Baked Ham
Buttered Parsley
Potatoes
Lima Beans in
Tomato Sauce
Red Apple, Banana
and Peanut Salad
Rolls, graham
Butter or Margarine
Cherry Tapioca Pudding
Beverage(s)

SUPPER
Consomme
Tomato Stuffed with
Shrimp Salad
Sesame Seed Rolls
Butter or Margarine
Coconut Cream Pie
Beverage(s)

MONDAY

BREAKFAST
Chilled Fruit Juice
Assorted Cold Cereals
or
Wheatena, with Cream
Cheese Danish Roll
Butter or Margarine
Beverage(s)

DINNER
Panned Liver and
Onions
Mashed Potatoes
Whole Kernel Corn
Sliced Harvard Beets
Bread, white and dark
Butter or Margarine
Baked Apple/topping

Beverage(s)

SUPPER
Vegetable Soup
Cold Corned Beef Slices
Potato Salad
Wholewheat Bread
Butter or Margarine
Relishes—Olives—Pickles
Assortment of Fresh
Fruit
Beverage(s)

TUESDAY	WEDNESDAY

BREAKFAST
- Stewed Apricots
- Fried Egg
- Hickory Smoked
  Bacon
- Golden Toast
- Butter or Margarine,
  Jam
- Beverage(s)

DINNER
- Grilled Frankfurter
  on Toasted Roll
- Boston Baked Beans
- German Style
  Sauerkraut
- Applesauce—Cookies
- Beverage(s)

SUPPER
- Cream of Asparagus
  Soup
- Cheese Omelet
- Mixed Green Salad/
  dressing
- Bread, wholewheat
- Butter or Margarine
- Angel Food Cake
- Beverage(s)

BREAKFAST
- Chilled Pineapple Juice
- Assorted Cold Cereals
  or
- Oatmeal, with Cream
- Hot Rolls
- Butter or Margarine
- Jelly
- Beverage(s)

DINNER
- Beef Rump Roast
- Browned Potatoes
- Buttered Green Peas
- Hearts of Lettuce
  dressing
- Bread
- Butter or Margarine
- Walnut Chiffon Cake
  (grind the nuts)
- Beverage(s)

SUPPER
- Baked Macaroni and
  Cheese and Tomatoes

- Bread, white and dark
- Butter or Margarine
- Mixed Vegetable Salad/
  dressing
- Cheese Cake
- Beverage(s)

THURSDAY	FRIDAY

BREAKFAST
Grapefruit Sections,
   Grenadine
Poached Egg on
   Buttered Toast
Prune Danish Roll
Butter or Margarine
Beverage(s)

BREAKFAST
Chilled Prune Juice
Old Fashioned Waffles
Honey Butter
Warm Maple Syrup
Beverage(s)

DINNER
Breaded Pork
   Tenderloin
Scalloped Potatoes

Buttered Asparagus
Cranberry, Jellied
Rolls
Butter or Margarine
Chocolate Chip Cookies
Beverage(s)

DINNER
Baked Pike Fillets
Lyonnaise Potatoes
Buttered Mixed
   Vegetables
Pimiento Cheese Stuffed
   Celery
Rolls
Butter or Margarine
Chilled Pears
Beverage(s)

SUPPER
Tomato Bouillon
Corned Beef Hash Patty
Home Fried Potatoes
Heated Rolls
Butter or Margarine
Cabbage and Apple
   Salad
Chilled Pineapple
   Chunks
Beverage(s)

SUPPER
Creamy Potato
   Soup
Salmon Salad
Lettuce Wedges/
   Russian Dressing

Bread, wholewheat
Butter or Margarine
Apple Brown Betty
   Orange Sauce
Beverage(s)

SATURDAY

BREAKFAST
  Chilled Fresh
    Melon Slice
  Assorted Cold Cereals
       or
  Cream of Wheat,
    warm milk
  Blueberry Muffin
  Butter or Margarine
  Beverage(s)

DINNER
  Salisbury Steak, with
    brown sauce
  Mashed Potatoes
  Baked Corn and Tomatoes
  Wilted Lettuce and Bacon
    Salad
  Rolls
  Butter or Margarine
  Fruit Cup
  Beverage(s)

SUPPER
  Celery Soup
  Hot Bologna-Holland
    Style
  Old Fashioned Sour
    Black Bread
  Butter or Margarine
  Green Beans
  Mustard—Horseradish
  Cream Puffs
  Beverage(s)

34th Week

SUNDAY	MONDAY
BREAKFAST	**BREAKFAST**

<table>
<tr><td>

BREAKFAST
Chilled Melon
Scrambled Eggs
Hickory Smoked
  Bacon
Raisin Toast
Butter or Margarine
Beverage(s)

DINNER
 Roast Tom Turkey
  and Dressing
Giblet Gravy
Mashed Potatoes
Buttered Brussel
  Sprouts
Fruit Salad, garnished
  with mint sprig
Rolls
Butter or Margarine
Baked Meringue with
  strawberries and
  topping
Beverage(s)

SUPPER
 V-8 Juice
Ham and Cheese
  Sandwiches
Sliced Tomato and
  Lettuce Salad
Chocolate Cookies,
  Ice Cream
Beverage(s)

</td><td>

BREAKFAST
Assorted Fruit Juices
Selected Cold Cereals
  or
Oatmeal, with cream
Toast, buttered
Jelly
Beverage(s)

DINNER
Cubed Steak
Egg Plant, oven fried

Buttered Green Peas
Shredded Lettuce
  with dressing
Bread, white and dark
Butter or Margarine
Spice Cake/Topping
Beverage(s)

SUPPER
Swedish Soup
Creamed Eggs and
  Cheese on Toasted
  English Muffins
Orange and Apple
  Salad
Extra Muffins with
  Butter or Margarine
Fresh Fruit (Apples,
  Bananas, Grapes)
Beverage(s)

</td></tr>
</table>

TUESDAY

BREAKFAST
  Orange Sections
  Poached Egg on
    Buttered Toast
  Hot Rolls
  Butter or Margarine
  Jam
  Beverage(s)

DINNER
  Corned Beef and
    Cabbage
  Boiled Potatoes
  Buttered coin sized
    Carrots
  Rye Bread, White
    Bread
  Butter or Margarine
  Gingerbread with
    Topping
  Beverage(s)

SUPPER
  Minestrone Soup

  Spaghetti with Tomato
    Meat Sauce
  Buttered Green Beans
  Tossed Green Salad/
    Dressing
  Canned Plums
  Jam Crunchies
    (cookies)
  Beverage(s)

WEDNESDAY

BREAKFAST
  Bananas with Cream
  Golden French Toast
  Maple Syrup or Honey
  Canadian Bacon
  Beverage(s)

DINNER
  Oven Fried Calves
    Liver with Bacon

  Buttered Parsley
    Potatoes
  Stewed Tomatoes and
    Celery
  Bread, white and dark
  Butter or Margarine
  Frosted Yellow Cake
    Squares
  Beverage(s)

SUPPER
  Corn Chowder
  Grilled Frankfurter on
    Hot Bun
  Baked Beans
  Cabbage-Apple-Celery
    Salad
  Chilled Pears
  Beverage(s)

THURSDAY	FRIDAY
BREAKFAST	**BREAKFAST**

BREAKFAST

Assorted Juices
Selected Cold Cereal
    or
Wheatena, with Cream
Plain Doughnuts
Butter or Margarine
Beverage(s)

DINNER

Meat Patties (Beef,
    Lamb,   Veal)
Hashed Brown
    Potatoes
Buttered Cauliflower
Hearts of Lettuce
    with Dressing
Rolls, cloverleaf
Butter or Margarine
Home-made Cottage
    Pudding
Beverage(s)

SUPPER

Cream of Tomato
    Soup
Creamed Chipped Beef
Hot Cornbread Squares

Jellied Peach Salad
White Cake with Boiled
    Chocolate Frosting

Beverage(s)

BREAKFAST

Grapefruit Half
Fried Egg
Plantation Sausage
Toast
Butter or Margarine,
    Jam
Beverage(s)

DINNER

Apricot Nectar
Deep Fried Scallops

Potatoes au Gratin

Buttered Lima Beans
Tomato Aspic
Rolls
Butter or Margarine
Vanilla Pudding
Beverage(s)

SUPPER

Clam Chowder with
    Saltines
Creamed Tuna with
    Cheese on Hot
    Buttered Baking
    Powder Biscuit (3)
Spinach with Butter
    Sauce
Chilled Fruit Cup
Beverage(s)

SATURDAY

BREAKFAST
  Assorted Juices
  Buttermilk Pancakes
  Honey Butter
  Warm Maple Syrup
  Grilled Ham
  Beverage(s)

DINNER
  Turkey Croquettes
  Cream Sauce
  Steamed Buttered Rice
  Buttered Peas
  Apricot and Banana
    Salad
  Hot Rolls
  Butter or Margarine
  Apple Sauce and
    Raisin Cake
  Beverage(s)

SUPPER
  Chicken Rice
    Soup
  Sliced Corned Beef
    Sandwich on Whole
    Wheat Bread
  Sliced Cucumber
    Salad
  Dill Pickles
  Fruit Gelatin
  Beverage(s)

35th Week

SUNDAY	MONDAY

BREAKFAST
- Chilled Orange Juice
- Country Fresh Egg
- Grilled Sausages
- Jelly Doughnuts
- Beverage(s)

BREAKFAST
- Fruit in Season
- Old Fashioned Waffles
- Crisp Bacon
- Honey or Maple Syrup
- Soft Butter
- Beverage(s)

DINNER
- Beef Roast
- Oven Browned
  Potatoes
- Mixed Vegetables
- Tomato and Lettuce
  Salad/dressing
- Rolls
- Butter or Margarine
- Peach Shortcake/
  Topping
- Beverage(s)

DINNER
- Baked Meat Loaf
  with Tomato Sauce

- Fluffy Mashed Potatoes
- Baked Squash with
  Brown Sugar
- Jellied Carrot and
  Pineapple Salad
- Muffins
- Butter or Margarine
- Lemon Chiffon Pie
- Beverage(s)

SUPPER
- Chicken Rice
  Soup
- Virginia Ham Sandwich
- Mustard and Catsup—
  Pickles
- Stuffed Celery
- Assorted Fresh Fruits
  (Apples, Grapes,
  Plums, Bananas)
- Beverage(s)

SUPPER
- Boston Baked Beans
  with Pork
- Grilled Weiners
- Warm Weiner Rolls
- Catsup—Mustard—
  Pickles
- Ice Cream—Cookies
- Beverage(s)

TUESDAY

BREAKFAST
Assorted Juices
Poached Egg on
Buttered Toast
Orange Danish Roll
Butter or Margarine
Jelly
Beverage(s)

DINNER
Broiled Ham Steak
Candied Sweet
Potatoes
Buttered Cauliflower
Bread, white and dark
Butter or Margarine
Malaga Grapes and
Orange Salad
Lemon Bread Pudding

Beverage(s)

SUPPER
Green Split Pea
Soup
Veal Salad Sandwich
Pear and Cottage
Cheese Salad
Bread, white and dark
Butter or Margarine
Cantaloupe
Beverage(s)

WEDNESDAY

BREAKFAST
Half Grapefruit
Selected Cold Cereal
or
Cream of Wheat, with
Cream
Golden Toast
Butter or Margarine
Jelly
Beverage(s)

DINNER
Braised Calves Liver
and Onions
Whipped Potatoes
Buttered Peas
Mixed Fruit Salad/
dressing
Bread, white and dark
Butter or Margarine
Vanilla Cookies
Beverage(s)

SUPPER
Tomato Rice Soup

Baked Corned Beef
Hash
Pineapple Cabbage
Slaw
Bread
Butter or Margarine
Tapioca Pudding with
Cherries
Beverage(s)

THURSDAY	FRIDAY

BREAKFAST
- Chilled Fruit Juice
- Buttermilk Pancakes
- Soft Butter
- Warm Maple Syrup
  - or Honey
- Beverage(s)

BREAKFAST
- Orange Slices
- Scrambled Eggs
- Crisp Bacon
- Toast
- Butter or Margarine
- Jelly
- Beverage(s)

DINNER
- Roast Loin of
  - Pork
- Fluffy Whipped Potatoes
- Sage Dressing
- Broccoli, with drawn
  - butter
- Applesauce
- Rolls, small
- Butter or Margarine
- Raspberry Sherbet
- Beverage(s)

DINNER
- Fried Fillet of Perch
  - with Tartar Sauce

- Parsley Buttered Potato
- Stewed Tomatoes
- Cucumber Watercress
  - Salad   with
  - Sour Cream
  - Dressing
- Bread, wholewheat
- Butter or Margarine
- Lemon Pie
- Beverage(s)

SUPPER
- Creamed Chicken
  - and Pimiento on
  - Toast
- Asparagus
- Sliced Orange Salad/
  - dressing
- Ginger Cookies,
  - homemade
- Beverage(s)

SUPPER
- Cream of Celery
  - Soup
- Grilled Cheese Sand-
  - wich
- Cabbage and Green
  - Pepper Salad
- Pound Cake
- Beverage(s)

SATURDAY

BREAKFAST
Stewed Prunes,
    Lemon Slices
Assorted Cold Cereals
    or
Oatmeal, with cream
Orange Danish Roll
Butter or Margarine
Beverage(s)

DINNER
Baked Thuringer
    Sausages and
    Sauerkraut
Parsley Buttered Potatoes
Black Bread (old fashioned)
Butter or Margarine
Jellied Fruit Salad
Baked Custard
Beverage(s)

SUPPER
Cream of Spinach
    Soup
Tomato, Lettuce and
    Bacon Sandwich on
    wholewheat bread
Chilled Strawberry Rhubarb
    Sauce
Cupcakes
Beverage(s)

36th Week

### SUNDAY	### MONDAY

BREAKFAST
Grapefruit and
    Orange Sections
Bacon Omelet
Golden Toast
Butter or Margarine
Jam or Marmalade
Beverage(s)

BREAKFAST
Chilled Fruit Juice
Assorted Cold Cereals
    or
Wheatena, with cream
Cheese Danish Roll
Butter or Margarine
Beverage(s)

DINNER
Roast Chicken
    Dressing
Giblet Gravy
Mashed Potatoes
Cauliflower with
    Cheese Sauce
Jellied Cranberry Salad
Rolls
Butter or Margarine
Meringue Shells
    Ice Cream—Fresh
    Strawberries
Beverage(s)

DINNER
Pot Roast and Gravy

Egg Noodles in
    Casserole
French Fried Onion
    Rings
Grapefruit Sections
    on Lettuce/Poppy
    Seed dressing
Apricot Upside-Down
    Cake
Beverage(s)

SUPPER
Vegetable Soup
Chef's Salad Bowl

Potato Chips
Sliced Tomatoes
Pickles
Bread, wholewheat
Butter or Margarine
Home-made Ginger
    Cookies
Beverage(s)

SUPPER
Hot Chicken a la King
    on Toast
Buttered Green Peas
Cole Slaw
Chilled Purple Plums,
    canned
Beverage(s)

TUESDAY	WEDNESDAY

BREAKFAST
Stewed Apricots
Fried Egg
Hickory Smoked Baocn
Golden Toast
Butter or Margarine
Jam
Beverage(s)

BREAKFAST
Chilled Pineapple Juice
Assorted Cold Cereals
or
Oatmeal, with cream
Hot Rolls
Butter or Margarine
Jelly
Beverage(s)

DINNER
Veal Roast
Duchess Potatoes
Broccoli Spears
Pineapple-Cottage
  Cheese-Cherry
  Salad
Rolls
Butter or Margarine
Molasses Cookies
Beverage(s)

DINNER
Baked Breaded
  Pork Chops
Baked Rice
Buttered Wax Beans
Bibb Lettuce Salad/
  dressing
Rolls
Butter or Margarine
Apple Pie
Beverage(s)

SUPPER
French Onion
  Soup
Sliced Roast Beef
  Sandwich
Catsup—Horseradish
Coin-Sized Buttered
  Carrots
Chocolate Cake
Beverage(s)

SUPPER
Tomato Bouillon

Peanut Butter and
  Bacon on Toast
Jellied Cream Cheese
  and Bing Cherry
  Salad
Bread Pudding with
  Lemon Sauce
Beverage(s)

THURSDAY	FRIDAY
BREAKFAST	**BREAKFAST**
Grapefruit Sections,	Chilled Prune Juice
Grenadine	Old Fashioned Waffles
Poached Egg on	Honey Butter
Buttered Toast	Warm Maple Syrup
Apple Danish Roll	Beverage(s)
Butter or Margarine	
Beverage(s)	
DINNER	**DINNER**
Italian Spaghetti with	Codfish Balls
Meat Sauce	Cream Sauce
Parmesan Cheese	Buttered Parsley Potatoes
Tossed Green Salad/	Harvard Beets
Italian dressing	Carrots and Cabbage
French Bread	Slaw
Garlic Butter or	Rolls
Butter or Margarine	Butter or Margarine
Ice Cream	Applesauce Cake
Beverage(s)	Beverage(s)
SUPPER	**SUPPER**
Corn Chowder and	Manhattan Clam
Saltines	Chowder
Hamburgers on Rolls	Macaroni and Cheese
Buttered Green Beans	
Potato Chips	Buttered Asparagus
Sweet Relish–Catsup	Bread, white and dark
Caramel Cake	Butter or Margarine
Beverage(s)	Fruit Cup
	Beverage(s)

SATURDAY

BREAKFAST
   Chilled Fresh Melon Slice
   Assorted Cold Cereals
       or
   Cream of Wheat,
     warm milk
   Cinnamon Raisin
     Pecan Roll
   Butter or Margarine
   Beverage(s)

DINNER
   Broiled Calves Liver
   Potatoes, Scalloped
   Shredded Cabbage
     Salad
   Buttered Broccoli
   Rolls
   Butter or Margarine
   Egg Nog Chiffon Pie
   Beverage(s)

SUPPER
   Baked Chicken Legs
   Country Fried Potatoes

   Glazed Carrots
   Bread, wholewheat
   Butter or Margarine
   Applesauce
   Beverage(s)

37th Week

SUNDAY	MONDAY
BREAKFAST	**BREAKFAST**
Chilled Melon	Assorted Fruit Juices
Scrambled Eggs	Selected Cold Cereals
Hickory Smoked	or
Bacon	Oatmeal, with cream
Plain Doughnut	Toast, Buttered
Beverage(s)	Jelly
	Beverage(s)
DINNER	**DINNER**
Apple Juice	Baked Meat Loaf,
Roast Leg of Veal	Mushroom Gravy
with Dressing	
Squash, brown	Country Fried
sugar sauce	Potatoes
Three-Bean Salad	Glazed Whole Carrots
Rolls	
Butter or Margarine	Wholewheat Rolls
Apricot Pie	Butter or Margarine
Beverage(s)	White Cake with
	Chocolate Frost-
	ing
	Beverage(s)
SUPPER	**SUPPER**
Chicken Noodle Soup	Barbecued Hamburgers
Jellied Waldorf Salad	on Toasted Buns
/Honey Fruited	Coleslaw
Dressing	Relishes—Pickles
Hot Pan Rolls	Blueberry Cobbler
Butter or Margarine	Beverage(s)
Baked Custard	
Beverage(s)	

TUESDAY	WEDNESDAY

BREAKFAST
Orange Sections
Poached Egg on
   Buttered Toast
Hot Rolls
Butter or Margarine
Jam
Beverage(s)

DINNER
Breaded Veal Cutlet
Baked Potato
Buttered Spinach
Fruit Salad with
   Stuffed Prunes/
   dressing
Bread—Butter or Margarine
Butterscotch Cookies
Beverage(s)

SUPPER
Chicken Broth
Individual Beef Pies
Jellied Peach and
   Cottage Cheese
   Salad
Rolls
Butter or Margarine
Floating Island Pudding
Beverage(s)

BREAKFAST
Bananas with Cream
Golden French Toast
Maple Syrup or Honey
Canadian Bacon
Beverage(s)

DINNER
Beef Stroganoff
Oven Browned
   Potatoes
Green Beans, French
   Style
Cabbage Salad
Rolls
Butter or Margarine
Chilled Apricots
Beverage(s)

SUPPER
Chicken Noodle Soup
Creamed Tuna-Egg
   Casserole
Cherry Red Fruit
   Gelatin
Jiffy Sponge Cake
Beverage(s)

THURSDAY	FRIDAY

BREAKFAST
Assorted Juices
Selected Cold Cereal
or
Wheatena, with cream
Corn Muffins
Butter or Margarine
Jelly
Beverage(s)

DINNER
Pork Chops in Sour
Cream
Baked Sweet Potatoes
Buttered Corn and
Green Peppers,
sauteed
Orange and Grapefruit
Salad
Currant Muffins
Butter or Margarine
Baked Apple/Topping

Beverage(s)

SUPPER
Cream of Lima Bean
Soup
Sliced Tongue
Sandwiches
(wholewheat)
Catsup—Horseradish
French Fried Egg
Plant (Cubed)
Jellied Fruit Salad

Vanilla Pinwheel
Cookies
Beverage(s)

BREAKFAST
Grapefruit Half
Fried Egg
Plantation Sausage
Toast
Butter or Margarine
Jam
Beverage(s)

DINNER
Baked Salmon Steak
with Tartar Sauce

Potatoes au Gratin
Sliced Tomato and
Lettuce Salad
Parsley Buttered Celery
and Carrots
Rolls
Butter or Margarine
Oatmeal Cookies
Beverage(s)

SUPPER
New England Clam
Chowder
Grilled Cheese
Sandwich
Jellied Pineapple and
Carrot Salad
Escalloped Apples

Beverage(s)

SATURDAY

BREAKFAST
  Assorted Juices
  Buttermilk Pancakes
  Honey Butter
  Warm Maple Syrup
  Grilled Ham
  Beverage(s)

DINNER
  Barbecued Pork Chops
  Baked Rice
  Creamed Cabbage
  Spring Garden Salad

  Rolls
  Butter or Margarine
  Strawberry Pie
  Beverage(s)

SUPPER
  Beef Broth with
    Barley
  Bologna, Holland Style
  Wholewheat Bread
  Butter or Margarine
  Mustard—Catsup—
    Horseradish
  Perfection Salad
    Squares
  Pineapple Upside Down
    Cake
  Beverage(s)

38th Week

SUNDAY	MONDAY

BREAKFAST
Chilled Orange Juice
Country Fresh Egg
Grilled Sausages
Coconut Doughnuts

Butter or Margarine
Beverage(s)

BREAKFAST
Fruit in Season
Old Fashioned Waffles
Crisp Bacon
Honey or Maple Syrup
Soft Butter
Beverage(s)

DINNER
Roast Chicken
Giblet Gravy
Bread Stuffing
Cranberry Sauce
Buttered Asparagus
Rolls, Hot Parker
House
Butter or Margarine
Ice Cream with
Chocolate Sauce
Beverage(s)

DINNER
Salisbury Steak with
Mushroom Sauce
Baked Potato
Whole Kernel Corn
Tomato and Lettuce
Salad
Bread, white and dark
Butter or Margarine
Whipped Fruit Gelatin
Beverage(s)

SUPPER
Cream of Mushroom
Soup
Cold Plate—Sliced Ham,
Cheese
Potato Salad
Pickled Beets
Bread, wholewheat
Butter or Margarine
Banana Cake
Beverage(s)

SUPPER
Split Pea Soup
Ham Sandwich on
Wholewheat Bread
Pickles and Olives
Cottage Cheese-Pine-
apple Salad
Refrigerator Cookies

Beverage(s)

TUESDAY	WEDNESDAY

BREAKFAST
  Assorted Juices
  Poached Egg on
    Buttered Toast
  Pineapple Danish Roll
  Butter or Margarine
  Beverage(s)

BREAKFAST
  Half Grapefruit
  Selected Cold Cereal
    or
  Cream of Wheat, with
    Cream
  Golden Toast
  Butter or Margarine
  Jelly
  Beverage(s)

DINNER
  Meat Loaf with
    Spanish Sauce
  Oven Browned
    Potatoes
  Peas, buttered
  Carrot, Prune and
    Celery Salad
  Peach Cobbler
  Beverage(s)

DINNER
  Vegetable Juice
  Chop Suey with Rice
  Baked Tomato with
    Crumb Topping
  Three-Bean Salad
  Rolls
  Butter or Margarine
  Graham Cracker Date
    Roll/Topping
  Beverage(s)

SUPPER
  Cream of Celery
    Soup
  Rice and Cheese
    Casserole
  Buttered Broccoli
  Deviled Egg Salad
  Vanilla Cream Pudding
    with Grated Orange
    Rind
  Beverage(s)

SUPPER
  Beef Noodle Soup
  Pork Link Sausages
    with Apple Rings
  Hashed Brown
    Potatoes
  Creamed Carrots
  Blue Plums, canned
  Beverage(s)

THURSDAY	FRIDAY

BREAKFAST
Chilled Fruit Juice
Buttermilk Pancakes
Soft Butter
Warm Maple Syrup
   or Honey
Beverage(s)

BREAKFAST
Orange Slices
Scrambled Eggs
Crisp Bacon
Toast
Butter or Margarine
Jelly
Beverage(s)

DINNER
Italian Spaghetti
   with Meat Sauce

Parmesan Cheese
Apple Gelatin with
   Crushed Pineapple
   Salad
Rolls
Butter or Margarine
Lemon Chiffon Pie
Beverage(s)

DINNER
Fried Fillet of Haddock,
   Lemon Wedges
Baked Potato
Stewed Tomatoes with
   Onion
Corn Muffin
Butter or Margarine—
   Apple Butter
Baked Custard
Beverage(s)

SUPPER
V-8 Juice
Toasted Chicken
   Salad Sandwiches
Celery Sticks
Carrot Sticks
Chocolate Cake with
   White Frosting
   (squares)
Beverage(s)

SUPPER
Cream of Celery
   Soup
Baked Salmon Loaf
Buttered Frenched
   Green Beans
Waldorf Salad
Bread
Butter or Margarine
Chilled Butterscotch
   Pudding
Beverage(s)

SATURDAY

BREAKFAST
Stewed Prunes,
    Lemon Slices
Assorted Cold Cereals
        or
Oatmeal, with cream
Lemon Danish
Butter or Margarine
Beverage(s)

DINNER
Tomato Juice
Pan Broiled Liver
    and Gravy
Mashed Potatoes
Asparagus Spears
    with Lemon Butter
Pear Halves on Lettuce/
    dressing
Rolls, wholewheat
Butter or Margarine
Molasses Bars
    (cookies)
Beverage(s)

SUPPER
Beef Broth and Rice
Knockwurst—Catsup
    and Horseradish
Baked Beans
Coleslaw
Bread, white and dark
Butter or Margarine
Chocolate Chiffon
    Cake
Beverage(s)

39th Week

SUNDAY

BREAKFAST
Grapefruit and
Orange Sections
Bacon Omelet
Golden Toast
Butter or Margarine
Jam or Marmalade
Beverage(s)

DINNER
Baked Ham
Buttered Parsley
Potatoes
Buttered Brussel
Sprouts
Fruit Salad/
dressing
Bread, wholewheat
Butter or Margarine
Coconut Custard Pie

Beverage(s)

SUPPER
Turkey Soup with
Rice
Veal Salad Plate
Potato Chips
Olives, Pickles and
Celery Curls
Rolls
Butter or Margarine
Vanilla Ice Cream
with Chocolate
Topping
Beverage(s)

MONDAY

BREAKFAST
Chilled Fruit Juice
Assorted Cold Cereals
or
Wheatena, with cream
Blueberry Muffin
Butter or Margarine
Beverage(s)

DINNER
Roast Shoulder of
Rolled Lamb, Mint
Jelly
Lyonnaise Potatoes

Fritter Fried Egg Plant
Rolls
Butter or Margarine
Carrots and Pineapple
Salad
Vanilla Cream Pudding
Beverage(s)

SUPPER
Cream of Celery Soup

Frankfurter on Toasted
Bun, buttered
Catsup—Relish—Mustard
Cabbage Salad
Orange Gelatin
Cubes—Cookies
Beverage(s)

TUESDAY	WEDNESDAY

BREAKFAST
- Stewed Apricots
- Fried Egg
- Hickory Smoked Bacon
- Golden Toast
- Butter or Margarine
- Jam
- Beverage(s)

BREAKFAST
- Chilled Pineapple Juice
- Assorted Cold Cereals
  - or
- Oatmeal, with cream
- Hot Rolls
- Butter or Margarine
- Jelly
- Beverage(s)

DINNER
- Veal Cutlets with Brown Gravy
- Mashed Potatoes
- Cucumber Salad
- Fried Parsnips
- Rolls, wholewheat
- Butter or Margarine— Jelly
- Cherry Upside Down Cake
- Beverage(s)

DINNER
- Spareribs and Sauerkraut
- Boiled Potatoes
- Beet and Cucumber Salad
- Corn Bread Muffins

- Butter or Margarine— Apple Butter
- Caramel Custard
- Beverage(s)

SUPPER
- Shepherd's Pie (cubed Lamb, Onions, Tomatoes, Parsley, Potatoes)
- Jellied Lime and Pear Salad
- Bread, white and dark
- Butter or Margarine
- Apricot Tapioca
- Beverage(s)

SUPPER
- Beef Noodle Soup
- Baked Hash
- Creamed Corn
- Cabbage and Apple Salad
- Angel Food Cake

- Beverage(s)

THURSDAY	FRIDAY

BREAKFAST
Grapefruit Sections,
   Grenadine
Poached Egg on
   Buttered Toast
Cranberry Nut Muffin
Butter or Margarine
Beverage(s)

BREAKFAST
Chilled Prune Juice
Old Fashioned Waffles
Honey Butter
Warm Maple Syrup
Beverage(s)

DINNER
Beef Stew (Onions,
   Potatoes, Carrots,
   Celery)
Jellied Citrus Fruit
   Salad
Bread, white and dark
Butter or Margarine—
   Jelly
Banana Cream Pie
Beverage(s)

DINNER
Shrimp Creole
Buttered Rice
Buttered Mixed
   Vegetables
Blushing Pear Salad
   with Peanut Butter
   Filling
Frosted Devils Food
   Cake
Beverage(s)

SUPPER
Navy Bean Soup

Boiled Ham Slices
Hashed Brown
   Potatoes
Tossed Salad
Rolls, homemade
Butter or Margarine
Chilled Pears
Beverage(s)

SUPPER
V-8 Juice
Canned Salmon Rice
   Loaf
Stewed Tomatoes

Tossed Green Salad

Corn Muffins
Butter or Margarine—
   Apple Butter
Prune Whip
Beverage(s)

SATURDAY

BREAKFAST
   Chilled Fresh
      Melon Slice
   Assorted Cold Cereals
         or
   Cream of Wheat,
      warm milk
   Pecan Roll
   Butter or Margarine
   Beverage(s)

DINNER
   Grilled Hamburger
   Cheese-Potato Casse-
      role
   Buttered Cauliflower
   Spiced Beet Salad/
      Sliced Eggs
   Rolled Wheat Muffin
   Butter or Margarine
   Cherry Gelatin/
      whipped Topping
   Beverage(s)

SUPPER
   Grapefruit Juice
   Pork Chop Suey with
      Chinese Noodles
   Rolls
   Butter or Margarine
   Cabbage-Pineapple
      Salad
   Chilled Plums
   Beverage(s)

40th Week

SUNDAY	MONDAY
BREAKFAST	**BREAKFAST**
Chilled Melon	Assorted Fruit Juices
Scrambled Eggs	Selected Cold Cereals
Hickory Smoked	or
Bacon	Oatmeal, with cream
Cinnamon Toast	Toast, Buttered
Butter or Margarine	Jelly
Beverage(s)	Beverage(s)
DINNER	**DINNER**
Roast Veal and Gravy	Baked Beans with
Fluffy Mashed Potatoes	1½ in. squares of
Buttered Broccoli	Ham
Perfection Salad/	Hot Potato Salad
Dressing	Carrot Sticks—Olives
Rolls, small	Boston Brown Bread
Pineapple Cream Pie	Butter or Margarine
Beverage(s)	Chilled Pears
	Beverage(s)
SUPPER	**SUPPER**
Cream of Corn Soup	Tomato Juice
	Beef Pot Pie,
Chicken Salad Sand-	Flaky Crust
wich (wholewheat	Peach and Cottage
bread)	Cheese Salad
Catsup—Mustard	Hot Parker House Rolls,
Potato Chips	homemade
Relish—Pickles	Butter or Margarine
Ice Cream	Cornflake Macaroons
Beverage(s)	
	Beverage(s)

TUESDAY

BREAKFAST
Orange Sections
Poached Egg on
   Buttered Toast
Hot Rolls
Butter or Margarine—
   Jam
Beverage(s)

DINNER
Hamburger Steaks
   with Tomato
   Sauce
Buttered Parsley Potatoes
Apple and Celery Salad

Scalloped Sweet Corn
Bread, wholewheat
Butter or Margarine
Snow Pudding Dessert
Beverage(s)

SUPPER
Apple Juice
Turkey a la king on
   Toast
Tossed Salad/
   dressing
Whipped Fruit
   Gelatin/Topping
Beverage(s)

WEDNESDAY

BREAKFAST
Bananas with Cream
Golden French Toast
Maple Syrup or Honey
Canadian Bacon
Beverage(s)

DINNER
Corned Beef and
   Cabbage
Boiled Potatoes,
   Buttered
Grated Carrot and
   Raisin Salad
Bread, wholewheat
Butter or Margarine
Chilled Slices of
   Pineapple
Old Fashioned Molasses
   Cookie
Beverage(s)

SUPPER
Vegetable Soup
Creamed Beef and
   Peas on Toast
Three Bean Salad
Applesauce
Beverage(s)

THURSDAY	FRIDAY

BREAKFAST
Assorted Juices
Selected Cold Cereal
or
Wheatena, with cream
Corn Muffins
Butter or Margarine—
Jelly
Beverage(s)

DINNER
Beef Roast and
Gravy
O'Brien Potatoes

Glazed Whole Carrots

Mixed Salad Greens/
Dressing
Rolls—Butter or
Margarine
Apple Pie with Streusel
Topping
Beverage(s)

SUPPER
Tomato Rice Soup

Mock Drum Sticks
(Veal and Pork)
Spinach with Bacon
Dressing
Bread—Butter or
Margarine
Chilled Queen Anne
Cherries
Beverage(s)

BREAKFAST
Grapefruit Half
Fried Egg
Plantation Sausage
Toast
Butter or Margarine—
Jam
Beverage(s)

DINNER
V-8 Juice
Baked Pike Fillets
French Fried Potatoes
Scalloped Celery and
Tomatoes
Creamy Cole Slaw

Rolls, wholewheat
Butter or Margarine
Chilled Purple Plums
Beverage(s)

SUPPER
Cream of Pea Soup,
Saltines
Individual Casseroles
of Cheese Fondue
Buttered Peas
Toasted Bread Squares
Butter or Margarine
Blueberry Cottage
Pudding, Lemon
Sauce
Beverage(s)

SATURDAY

BREAKFAST
    Assorted Juices
    Buttermilk Pancakes
    Honey Butter
    Warm Maple Syrup
    Grilled Ham
    Beverage(s)

DINNER
    Swedish Meat Balls
    Potatoes au Gratin

    Whole Kernel Corn
    Yankee Slaw (cabbage,
       carrots, green
       peppers)
    Bread, wholewheat
    Butter or Margarine
    Whipped Fruit
       Gelatin/Topping
    Beverage(s)

SUPPER
    Chicken Rice Soup

    Assorted Sandwiches
    Fruit Salad/Honey Fruit
       Dressing
    Chocolate Icebox Cake
    Beverage(s)

41st Week

SUNDAY

BREAKFAST
Chilled Orange Juice
Country Fresh Egg
Grilled Sausages
Cinnamon Doughnuts

Butter or Margarine
Beverage(s)

DINNER
Apple Juice
Young Roast Turkey
   Giblet Gravy

New England Bread
   Stuffing
Buttered Peas
Cranberry Sauce
Fruit Salad
Parker House Rolls

Butter or Margarine
Pineapple Sherbet
Beverage(s)

SUPPER
Macaroni-Ham-Cheese
   Casserole
Crisp Vegetable
   Salad
Pickles—Olives
Stuffed Celery
Red Cherry Tarts
Beverage(s)

MONDAY

BREAKFAST
Fruit in Season
Old Fashioned Waffles
Crisp Bacon
Honey or Maple Syrup
Soft Butter
Beverage(s)

DINNER
Tomato Juice
Baked Hash (including
   potatoes)
Creamed Style Corn
Cottage Cheese with
   Chopped Chives
Rolls
Butter or Margarine
Apple Dumpling
Beverage(s)

SUPPER
Swiss Steak
Buttered Broccoli Cuts
Hashed Brown
   Potatoes
Bread
Butter or Margarine
Grilled Tomatoes
Caramel Bavarian
Beverage(s)

TUESDAY	WEDNESDAY

BREAKFAST
  Assorted Juice
  Poached Egg on
    Buttered Toast
  Prune Danish Roll
  Butter or Margarine
  Jelly
  Beverage(s)

BREAKFAST
  Half Grapefruit
  Selected Cold Cereal
      or
  Cream of Wheat,
    with cream
  Golden Toast
  Butter or Margarine—
    Jelly
  Beverage(s)

DINNER
  Roast Pork
  Glazed Sweet
    Potatoes
  Green Beans, french style
  Fried Parsnips
  Graham Rolls
  Butter or Margarine
  Lemon Bread Pudding
  Beverage(s)

DINNER
  Veal Roast
  Buttered Rice
  Asparagus
    Hollandaise
  Molded Spiced Fruit
    Salad
  Orange Rolls
  Butter or Margarine
  Cherry Pie
  Beverage(s)

SUPPER
  Cream of Asparagus
    Soup
  Corn Fritters
  Maple Syrup (warm)
  Peach and Cottage
    Cheese Salad
  Orange Sherbet
  Beverage(s)

SUPPER
  Cream of Chicken
    Soup
  Stuffed Green Peppers
  Parsleyed Carrots
  Rolls
  Butter or Margarine
  Steamed Fig Pudding
  Beverage(s)

THURSDAY	FRIDAY
BREAKFAST	**BREAKFAST**
Chilled Fruit Juice	Orange Slices
Buttermilk Pancakes	Scrambled Eggs
Soft Butter	Crisp Bacon
Warm Maple Syrup	Toast
or Honey	Butter or Margarine
Beverage(s)	Jelly
	Beverage(s)
DINNER	**DINNER**
Ham Loaf	Baked Salmon Steak
with Horseradish	with Tartar Sauce
Sauce	
Buttered Potatoes	Oven Browned Potatoes
Southern Style Green	
Beans	Parsley Buttered Carrots
Head Lettuce	Jellied Vegetable Salad
Rouquefort Cheese	
Dressing	Corn Meal Muffins
Rolls, homemade	Butter or Margarine
Butter or Margarine	or Apple Butter
Apricot Pie	Baked Winesap Apple/
Beverage(s)	Topping
	Beverage(s)
SUPPER	**SUPPER**
Beef Bouillon	Cream of Celery Soup
Grilled Liver and	
Bacon (calves	Egg Salad Sandwiches
liver)	
Stewed Whole	Mixed Green Salad/
Tomatoes	French dressing
Shoestring Potatoes	
	Pineapple Cheese
Butter or Margarine	Cake
Chocolate Marsh-	Beverage(s)
mallow Squares	
Beverage(s)	

SATURDAY

BREAKFAST
Stewed Prunes,
Lemon Slices
Assorted Cold Cereals
or
Oatmeal, with cream
Cherry Danish
Butter or Margarine
Beverage(s)

DINNER
Baked Pork Chops
Applesauce
Cottage Fried
Potatoes
Cabbage au Gratin
Sliced Tomato on
Lettuce Salad/
dressing
Rolls, homemade
Butter or Margarine
Whipped Orange
Gelatin
Beverage(s)

SUPPER
Cream of Spinach
Soup
Corned Beef Sand-
wiches on Rye
Bread
Potato Chips
Celery and Carrot
Sticks
Dill Pickles
Peach Crumble
Dessert
Beverage(s)

42nd Week

SUNDAY

BREAKFAST
  Grapefruit and
    Orange Sections
  Bacon Omelet
  Golden Toast
  Butter or Margarine
  Jam or Marmalade
  Beverage(s)

DINNER
  Roast Leg of Lamb,
    Mint Jelly
  Mashed Sweet Potatoes
  Buttered Broccoli Spears
  Rolls, homemade
  Butter or Margarine
  Sliced Radishes and
    Lettuce/dressing
  Chocolate Souffle
    (baked in individual
    molds)
  Beverage(s)

SUPPER
  Chicken Noodle Soup
  Cold Plate (Boiled Ham,
    Swiss Cheese,
    Potato Salad
    Relishes—Green and
    Black Olives
  Bread, wholewheat
  Butter or Margarine
  Fresh Fruits (Apples,
    oranges, grapes,
    bananas)
  Beverage(s)

MONDAY

BREAKFAST
  Chilled Fruit Juice
  Assorted Cold Cereals
    or
  Wheatena, with cream
  Cheese Danish Roll
  Butter or Margarine
  Beverage(s)

DINNER
  V-8 Juice
  Creamed Chunks of
    Chicken
  Mashed Potatoes
  Asparagus
  Grapefruit—Malaga
    Grapes Salad/
    Honey Fruit
    Dressing
  Angel Food Cake/
    Topping
  Beverage(s)

SUPPER
  Split Pea Soup
  Oven Baked French
    Toast with Maple
    Syrup
  Pork Sausage Links
  Tossed Salad Greens/
    dressing
  Whipped Black Cherry
    Gelatin/topping
  Beverage(s)

TUESDAY	WEDNESDAY

BREAKFAST
- Stewed Apricots
- Fried Egg
- Hickory Smoked
  Bacon
- Golden Toast
- Butter or Margarine
- Jam
- Beverage(s)

DINNER
- Spanish Rice with
  Chopped Meat
- Shredded Cabbage,
  Apple and Ground
  Nut Salad
- Graham Rolls
- Butter or Margarine
- Pineapple Cream
  Pudding
- Beverage(s)

SUPPER
- Beef Noodle Soup
- Turkey Salad
- Fried Parsnips
- Sliced Tomato on
  Lettuce
- Corn Bread
- Butter or Margarine—
  Plum Butter
- Honey Bars (cookies)

- Beverage(s)

BREAKFAST
- Chilled Pineapple Juice
- Assorted Cold Cereals
  or
- Oatmeal, with cream
- Hot Rolls
- Butter or Margarine
- Jelly
- Beverage(s)

DINNER
- Chicken Rice Soup

- Beans and Sausage,
  Mexican Style
- Tossed Vegetable
  Salad
- Bread, black sour
  and white
- Butter or Margarine
- Chilled Purple Plums
- Beverage(s)

SUPPER
- Tomato Juice
- Salami and Liverwurst
  Sandwiches, with
  lettuce
- Jellied Fruit Salad

- Orange Bread Pudding,
  Orange Sauce
- Beverage(s)

THURSDAY	FRIDAY

BREAKFAST

Grapefruit Sections,
  Grenadine
Poached Egg on
  Buttered Toast
Apple Danish Roll
Butter or Margarine
Beverage(s)

BREAKFAST

Chilled Prune Juice
Old Fashioned Waffles
Honey Butter
Warm Maple Syrup
Beverage(s)

DINNER

Barbecued Hamburger
  Steak
French Fried Potatoes
Squash
Buttered Beets
Hot Baking Powder
  Biscuits
Butter or Margarine
Catsup—Apple Butter
Custard
Beverage(s)

DINNER

Creamed Codfish and
  Hard-Cooked Eggs
  on Boiled Potato
Buttered Green Peas
Head Lettuce/Thous-
  and Island Dressing

Rolls
Butter or Margarine
Chilled Peaches
Beverage(s)

SUPPER

Vegetable Soup
Sliced Corned Beef
  Sandwiches
Potato Salad
Jellied Vegetable
  Salad
Homemade Roll
Boston Cream Pie
Beverage(s)

SUPPER

Tuna Noodle Casserole
Buttered Asparagus
  Spears
Bread, white and dark
Butter or Margarine
Whipped Fruit Gelatin
Beverage(s)

SATURDAY

BREAKFAST
    Chilled Fresh Melon Slice
    Assorted Cold Cereals
        or
    Cream of Wheat, warm
      milk
    Pineapple Muffins
    Butter or Margarine
    Beverage(s)

DINNER
    Pork Roast
    Mashed Squash
    Creamed Cauliflower
      with Pimiento Strips
    Grapefruit and Orange
      Sections on Curly
      Endive/French
      Dressing
    Rolls
    Butter or Margarine
    Applesauce Cake
    Beverage(s)

SUPPER
    V-8 Juice
    Knockwurst and
      Sauerkraut
    Buttered Peas
    Bread, white and dark
    Butter or Margarine
    Grape Gelatin Squares
    Beverage(s)

43rd Week

SUNDAY	MONDAY

BREAKFAST
  Chilled Melon
  Scrambled Eggs
  Hickory Smoked
    Bacon
  Cinnamon Raisin
    Pecan Rolls
  Beverage(s)

BREAKFAST
  Assorted Fruit Juices
  Selected Cold Cereals
    or
  Oatmeal, with cream
  Toast, buttered
  Jelly
  Beverage(s)

DINNER
  Southern Fried
    Chicken
  Cream Gravy
  Mashed Potatoes
  Buttered Peas and
    Carrots
  Cranberry and
    Orange Salad
  Rolls
  Butter or Margarine
  Raspberry Sherbet
  Beverage(s)

DINNER
  Irish Lamb Stew with
    Dumplings
  Buttered Frozen Peas
    with Mushrooms
  Pineapple and Melon
    Salad/Celery Seed
    Fruit Dressing
  Rolls, wholewheat
  Butter or Margarine
  Cornflake Kisses
  Beverage(s)

SUPPER
  Tomato Bouillon
  Cheeseburger
  Potato Chips
  Sliced Tomato on
    Lettuce Leaf
  Chocolate Custard Pie
  Beverage(s)

SUPPER
  Consomme
  Chicken Salad on
    Lettuce
  Bread, white and dark
  Butter or Margarine
  Jellied Vegetables
    (Salad)
  Chocolate Tapioca
    Cream Pudding
  Beverage(s)

| TUESDAY | WEDNESDAY |

BREAKFAST
  Orange Sections
  Poached Egg on
    Buttered Toast
  Hot Rolls
  Butter or Margarine
  Jam
  Beverage(s)

BREAKFAST
  Bananas with Cream
  Golden French Toast
  Maple Syrup or Honey
  Canadian Bacon
  Beverage(s)

DINNER
  Pork Noodle Casserole
  Buttered Spinach with
    Bacon Bits
  Cabbage and Pineapple
    Salad
  Bread, white and dark
  Butter or Margarine
  White Grapes
  Beverage(s)

DINNER
  Breaded Veal Cutlet

  Parsley Creamed
    Potatoes
  Buttered Asparagus
  Tossed Vegetable
    Salad
  Rolls, homemade
  Butter or Margarine
  Mocha Almond
    Frozen Pie
  Beverage(s)

SUPPER
  Corn Chowder
  Sliced Corned Beef
    Sandwich, (whole-
    wheat bread)
  Baked Squash with
    brown sugar
  Snow Pudding, cut in
    squares and served
    with Custard Sauce
  Beverage(s)

SUPPER
  Vegetable Broth
  Eggs Benedict (poached
    egg on ½ buttered
    english muffin with
    mock hollandaise
    sauce
  Buttered Green Peas
  Waldorf Salad
  Cupcakes
  Beverage(s)

THURSDAY	FRIDAY
BREAKFAST	**BREAKFAST**
Assorted Juices	Grapefruit Half
Selected Cold Cereal	Fried Egg
or	Plantation Sausage
Wheatena, with Cream	Toast
Corn Muffins	Butter or Margarine
Butter or Margarine	Jam
Jelly	Beverage(s)
Beverage(s)	
DINNER	**DINNER**
Meat Loaf,	Fried Yellow Perch
Gravy	with Tartar Sauce
Buttered Boiled	
Potatoes	Baked Potato
Scalloped Corn	Broccoli Polonaise
Head Lettuce Wedges/	Pear with Shredded
dressing	Cheese on Lettuce
Rolls	Leaf/dressing
Butter or Margarine	Bran Rolls
Yellow Cake with	Butter or Margarine
Chocolate Icing	Pineapple Cheese
Beverage(s)	Cake
	Beverage(s)
SUPPER	**SUPPER**
Vegetable Soup	Cream of Tomato
Mock Chicken Legs	Soup
Hashed Brown	Tunafish Salad
Potatoes	Bread, white and dark
Glazed Carrots, coin	Butter or Margarine
sized	Potato Chips
Bread, white and dark	Sliced Beet and Onion
Butter or Margarine	Salad
Baked Custard	Apple Crisp
Beverage(s)	Beverage(s)

SATURDAY

BREAKFAST
  Assorted Juices
  Buttermilk Pancakes
  Honey Butter
  Warm Maple Syrup
  Grilled Ham
  Beverage(s)

DINNER
  Baked Meat Pie
      (including carrots,
      onions, potatoes)

  Jellied Fruit Salad
  Rolls, homemade
  Vanilla Ice Cream
  Beverage(s)

SUPPER
  Chicken Noodle Soup
  Grilled Frankfurter on
      Hot Roll
  Mustard—Catsup—Relish
  Potato Salad
  Bread, white and dark
  Butter or Margarine
  Cottage Cheese and
      Chives Salad
  Raisin Cake with
      Lemon Frosting
  Beverage(s)

44th Week

SUNDAY	MONDAY

BREAKFAST
  Chilled Orange Juice
  Country Fresh Egg
  Grilled Sausages
  Almond Nut
    Doughnuts
  Butter or Margarine
  Beverage(s)

BREAKFAST
  Fruit in Season
  Old Fashioned Waffles
  Crisp Bacon
  Honey or Maple Syrup
  Soft Butter
  Beverage(s)

DINNER
  Baked Ham with
    Honey Glaze
  Baked Sweet Potatoes
    with butter
  Buttered Baby Lima
    Beans
  Raspberry Ring Salad
  Vienna Bread
  Butter or Margarine
  Vanilla Ice Cream
  Beverage(s)

DINNER
  Chunks of Chicken
    with Dumplings
  Buttered Julienne
    Green Beans
  Chef's Salad/French
    Dressing
  Bread, white and dark
  Butter or Margarine
  Baked Coconut
    Custard
  Beverage(s)

SUPPER
  Tomato Rice Soup

  Ham Sandwiches (whole-
    wheat bread)
  Celery Sticks
  Blond Brownies
  Beverage(s)

SUPPER
  Split Pea Soup
    Saltines
  Baked Green Peppers
    (stuffed with ground
    meat, tomato sauce)
  Fresh Fruit Salad
  Bread
  Butter or Margarine
  Blueberry Cupcake
  Beverage(s)

TUESDAY

BREAKFAST
Assorted Juices
Poached Egg on
  Buttered Toast
Prune Danish Roll
Butter or Margarine
Beverage(s)

DINNER
Stuffed Veal Shoulder
Bread Stuffing
Natural Gravy
Hashed Brown
  Potatoes
Buttered Cauliflower
Sliced Pineapple and
  Cream Cheese
  Salad
Rolls
Butter or Margarine
Nut and Raisin
  Cookies
Beverage(s)

SUPPER
Scotch Broth and
  Barley
Boston Baked Beans
  (with 1-in. chunks
  of ham)
Brown Bread
Butter or Margarine
Chilled Pineapple
Beverage(s)

WEDNESDAY

BREAKFAST
Half Grapefruit
Selected Cold Cereal
  or
Cream of Wheat,
  with cream
Golden Toast
Butter or Margarine
Jelly
Beverage(s)

DINNER
Oven Baked Pork Chops
Brown Rice with
  Mushroom Sauce
Buttered Green Peas
Jellied Carrot and
  Pineapple Salad
Rolls
Butter or Margarine
Cocoa Cupcakes
Beverage(s)

SUPPER
Beef Broth
Cold Sliced Beef Tongue
  Sandwich (wholewheat
  bread)
French Fried Potatoes
Cole Slaw
Wax Beans
Peanut Butter Cookies
Beverage(s)

THURSDAY	FRIDAY
BREAKFAST	**BREAKFAST**

THURSDAY

BREAKFAST
Chilled Fruit Juice
Buttermilk Pancakes
Soft Butter
Warm Maple Syrup
   or Honey
Beverage(s)

DINNER
Spareribs, barbecued

Boiled Potatoes
Braised Celery
Shredded Lettuce
   Salad/dressing
Bread, wholewheat
Butter or Margarine
Lemon Pie
Beverage(s)

SUPPER
Potato Soup
Frankfurter and
   Sauerkraut
Dark Mustard—Catsup—
   Horseradish
Fried Potatoes
Hot Spiced Beets
Bread, sour black and
   white
Butter or Margarine
Chocolate Cake Squares
   with White Icing
Beverage(s)

FRIDAY

BREAKFAST
Orange Slices
Scrambled Eggs
Crisp Bacon
Toast
Butter or Margarine—
   Jelly
Beverage(s)

DINNER
Scallops   with
   Tartar Sauce
Creamed Potatoes
   with Chives
Buttered Green Beans
   with Pimiento
   Strips
Mixed Green Salad/
   dressing
Rolls, homemade
Lemon Sherbet
Beverage(s)

SUPPER
V-8 Juice
Tuna Noodle Casserole
Asparagus, buttered

Bread, white and dark
Butter or Margarine
Date-Nut Squares
Beverage(s)

SATURDAY

BREAKFAST
Stewed Prunes, Lemon
Slices
Assorted Cold Cereals
or
Oatmeal, with cream
Cinnamon Streusel
Danish
Butter or Margarine
Beverage(s)

DINNER
Braised Beef
Minute Steak
Oven Browned Potatoes

Buttered Green Beans
Assorted Relish Tray
with Celery and
Green Olives
Rolls, homemade
Butter or Margarine
Home-Baked Fruit Pie

Beverage(s)

SUPPER
Vegetable Soup
Pork Link Sausages
with Apple Rings
Hashed Brown
Potatoes
Spinach, buttered
Bread, white and dark
Butter or Margarine
Purple Plums
Beverage(s)

45th Week

SUNDAY

BREAKFAST
  Grapefruit and
    Orange Sections
  Bacon Omelet
  Golden Toast
  Butter or Margarine
  Jam or Marmalade
  Beverage(s)

DINNER
  Country Fried Chicken,
    Cream Gravy
  Mashed Potatoes
  Spiced Peaches
  Whole Kernel Corn
  Pineapple-Melon-Apple
    Salad/Poppy Seed
    Fruit Dressing
  Rolls, homemade
  Butter or Margarine
  Vanilla Ice Cream/
    Chocolate Sauce
  Beverage(s)

SUPPER
  Turkey Soup
  Cold Plate (Ham Slices,
    Deviled Egg,
    Slice of Cheese)
  Bread, wholewheat and
    white
  Butter or Margarine
  Prune Spice Cake/
    Topping
  Beverage(s)

MONDAY

BREAKFAST
  Chilled Fruit Juice
  Assorted Cold Cereals
    or
  Wheatena, with cream
  Cherry Danish Roll
  Butter or Margarine
  Beverage(s)

DINNER
  Old Fashioned Baked
    Ham (with bone)

  Candied Sweet Potatoes

  Steamed Cabbage
  Pear and Shredded
    Cheese Salad
  Bread, white and dark
  Butter or Margarine
  Orange Tapioca Pudding
  Beverage(s)

SUPPER
  Grapefruit Juice
  Scrambled Eggs and
    Dried Beef
  Buttered Peas and
    Carrots
  Bread, white and dark
  Butter or Margarine
  Pineapple Upside
    Down Cake
  Beverage(s)

TUESDAY	WEDNESDAY

BREAKFAST
Stewed Apricots
Fried Egg
Hickory Smoked
  Bacon
Golden Toast
Butter or Margarine
Jam
Beverage(s)

DINNER
Beef Stew   and
  Dumplings
Jellied Citrus Salad/
  Fruit Salad Dressing
Bread, wholewheat
  and white
Butter or Margarine
Chilled Butterscotch
  Pudding
Beverage(s)

SUPPER
Cream of Mushroom
  Soup
Beef Patty on Ham-
  burger Roll
Potato Salad
Sliced Tomatoes
Onion and Pickle Slices
Strawberry Ice Cream
Beverage(s)

BREAKFAST
Chilled Pineapple Juice
Assorted Cold Cereals
  or
Oatmeal, with cream
Hot Rolls,
Butter or Margarine
Jelly
Beverage(s)

DINNER
Braised Beef/Brown
  Rice
Cabbage Slaw—
  Pimiento
Buttered June Peas
Rolls, wholewheat
Butter or Margarine
Chilled Peaches
Beverage(s)

SUPPER
Apple Juice
Cheese Vegetable Rare-
  bit on Toast, (includes
  cheese, onion, green
  peppers and celery)
Whole Kernel Corn
Prune Crunch/Topping
Beverage(s)

THURSDAY

BREAKFAST
Grapefruit Sections,
Grenadine
Poached Egg on
Buttered Toast
Apple Danish Roll
Butter or Margarine
Beverage(s)

DINNER
Liver Creole
Buttered Rice
Buttered Asparagus
Raisin Bread
Butter or Margarine
Pineapple Chunks
Beverage(s)

SUPPER
Chili Con Carne
Apple-Cabbage-Carrot
Slaw
Poppy Seed Hard Rolls
Butter or Margarine
Pumpkin Pie
Beverage(s)

FRIDAY

BREAKFAST
Chilled Prune Juice
Old Fashioned Waffles
Honey Butter
Warm Maple Syrup
Beverage(s)

DINNER
Baked Perch Fillets
with Fluffy Cheese
Sauce
Buttered Spinach
Boiled Parsley Potatoes
Bread
Butter or Margarine
Raisin Bread Pudding

Beverage(s)

SUPPER
Cream of Tomato
Soup
Tunafish Salad
French Fried Potatoes
Tossed Green Salad/
dressing
Bread, wholewheat,
white
Butter or Margarine
Yellow Cake with
White Frosting

Beverage(s)

SATURDAY

BREAKFAST
Chilled Fresh
Melon Slice
Assorted Cold Cereals
or
Cream of Wheat,
warm milk
Chocolate Coconut
Doughnut
Beverage(s)

DINNER
Ground Beef and
Spaghetti
Buttered Broccoli
Tossed Green Salad

French Bread
Butter or Margarine
Frosted Yellow Cup-
cake
Beverage(s)

SUPPER
Spinach Soup
Ham Sandwich (whole-
wheat or white bread)
Confetti Cole Slaw
Relish Tray
Apple Raisin Cobbler
Beverage(s)

46th Week

SUNDAY

BREAKFAST
  Chilled Melon
  Scrambled Eggs
  Hickory Smoked
    Bacon
  Surprise Muffins
  Butter or Margarine
  Beverage(s)

DINNER
  Roast Loin of
    Pork
  Baked Potato, butter
    or sour cream
  Green Beans,
    French Style
  Grapefruit and Orange
    Sections on Curly
    Endive/dressing
  Rolls, homemade
  Butter or Margarine
  Chocolate Pie
  Beverage(s)

SUPPER
  Tomato Bouillon with
    Rice
  Cold Plate—Ham, Cheese,
    Potato Salad
    Pickles, Olives, (green
    and black)
  Bread—white and dark
  Fresh Fruit
  Beverage(s)

MONDAY

BREAKFAST
  Assorted Fruit Juices
  Selected Cold Cereals
    or
  Oatmeal, with cream
  Toast, buttered
  Jelly
  Beverage(s)

DINNER
  Meat Loaf   Mush-
    room Gravy
  Baked Potato
  Buttered Spinach
  Cole Slaw (white and
    red cabbage)
  Biscuits, homemade
  Butter or Margarine
  Chilled Apricots
  Beverage(s)

SUPPER
  Carrot and Celery Soup
  Assorted Sandwiches
  Deviled Egg and
    Tomato Salad
  Applesauce
  Cookies
  Beverage(s)

TUESDAY

BREAKFAST
  Orange Sections
  Poached Egg on
    Buttered Toast
  Hot Rolls
  Butter or Margarine
  Jam
  Beverage(s)

DINNER
  Spareribs and
    Sauerkraut
  Boiled Potatoes
  Waldorf Salad on
    Lettuce
  Bread, white and dark
  Butter or Margarine
  Coconut Cookies
  Beverage(s)

SUPPER
  Tomato Juice
  Shepherd's Pie
    (includes onion,
    carrot, celery
    and potatoes)
  Pear in Lime Gelatin

  Rolls, graham
  Butter or Margarine
  Maple Nut Chiffon
    Cake
  Beverage(s)

WEDNESDAY

BREAKFAST
  Bananas with Cream
  Golden French Toast
  Maple Syrup or Honey
  Canadian Bacon
  Beverage(s)

DINNER
  Lamb Roast, Mint
    Jelly
  Mashed Sweet Potatoes
  Buttered Turnips
  Parkerhouse Rolls,
    homemade
  Butter or Margarine
  Pineapple and Carrot
    Salad
  Baked Apple/Topping
  Beverage(s)

SUPPER
  Barbecued Beef on
    Roll
  Escalloped Corn
  Cabbage and Green
    Pepper Slaw
  Baked Custard
  Beverage(s)

THURSDAY	FRIDAY

BREAKFAST
- Assorted Juices
- Selected Cold Cereal
  - or
- Wheatena, with cream
- Corn Muffins
- Butter or Margarine
- Jelly
- Beverage(s)

DINNER
- Creamed Chunks of
  - Chicken on Toast
- Asparagus Spears, buttered
- Tomato and Shredded
  - Lettuce/dressing
- Coconut Cream Pie
- Beverage(s)

SUPPER
- Vegetable Soup
- Beef Chop Suey—
  - Steamed Rice
- Bread, white and dark
- Butter or Margarine
- Chilled Pears
- Beverage(s)

BREAKFAST
- Grapefruit Half
- Fried Egg
- Plantation Sausage
- Toast
- Butter or Margarine—
  - Jam
- Beverage(s)

DINNER
- Scallops
  - Tartar Sauce
- Buttered Parsley
  - Potatoes
- Stewed Tomatoes/
  - croutons
- Shredded Lettuce
  - Salad/dressing
- Rolls
- Butter or Margarine
- Cookies
- Beverage(s)

SUPPER
- Puree of Pea Soup

- Grilled Cheese Sand-
  - wich
- Buttered Mixed Vege-
  - tables
- Apple Pie
- Beverage(s)

SATURDAY

BREAKFAST
  Assorted Juices
  Buttermilk Pancakes
  Honey Butter
  Warm Maple Syrup
  Grilled Ham
  Beverage(s)

DINNER
  Oven Fried Calves
    Liver
  Creamed New Potatoes
    and Peas
  Buttered Corn
  Banana-Grapefruit-Grape
    Salad/Honey Fruit
    Dressing
  Apricot Crisp
  Beverage(s)

SUPPER
  Tomato and Celery Soup
  Baked Beans/Sliced
    Frankfurters
  Tossed Green Salad
  Brown Bread—with Cream
    Cheese, if desired
  Butter or Margarine
  Fruit Cup
  Beverage(s)

47th Week

SUNDAY

BREAKFAST
Chilled Orange Juice
Country Fresh Egg
Grilled Sausages
Jelly Doughnuts
Beverage(s)

DINNER
Broiled Ham Steak
Scalloped Potatoes

Buttered Baby Whole
  Beets
Chilled Molded Fruit
  Salad
Rolls
Butter or Margarine
Mincemeat Pie
  (homemade)
Beverage(s)

SUPPER
Chili
Crackers
Corn Bread
Butter or Margarine,
  Apple Butter
Chilled Peaches
Beverage(s)

MONDAY

BREAKFAST
Fruit in Season
Old Fashioned Waffles
Crisp Bacon
Honey or Maple Syrup
Soft Butter
Beverage(s)

DINNER
Creamed Turkey
  Chunks, Pimiento
Parsley Buttered Rice
Buttered Peas and
  Carrots
Jellied Cranberry and
  Orange Salad
Rolls, homemade
Butter or Margarine—
  Jelly
Crispy Oatmeal
  Cookies
Beverage(s)

SUPPER
Cream of Spinach
  Soup
Cheese Omelet
Green Beans, French
  Style
Bread, white and dark
Butter or Margarine
Cottage Pudding
  with Lemon Sauce
Beverage(s)

TUESDAY	WEDNESDAY

BREAKFAST
- Assorted Juices
- Poached Egg on
  Buttered Toast
- Orange Pineapple
  Danish Roll
- Butter or Margarine—
  Jelly
- Beverage(s)

DINNER
- Sauteed Chicken Livers
- Creamed Potatoes
- Stewed Tomatoes
- Cottage Cheese and
  Chives Salad
- Fruit Cup
- Beverage(s)

SUPPER
- Corn Chowder
- Apple Fritters
- Warm Maple Syrup
- Romaine Lettuce—
  Grapefruit Sections
  with Sesame Seed
  Dressing
- Fruit Cake—Hard Sauce

- Beverage(s)

BREAKFAST
- Half Grapefruit
- Selected Cold Cereal
  or
- Cream of Wheat,
  with Cream
- Golden Toast
- Butter or Margarine
- Beverage(s)

DINNER
- Minute Steaks
- French Fried Potatoes
- Broccoli, buttered
- Carrot Sticks—Stuffed
  Celery
- Bread, white and dark
- Butter or Margarine
- Cherry Pie, homemade

- Beverage(s)

SUPPER
- Chicken Rice Soup
- Steamed Frankfurters
- Mustard
- Boston Baked Beans
- Bread, white and dark
- Butter or Margarine
- Hearts of Lettuce
  Thousand Island
  Dressing
- Jelly Roll, home baked
- Beverage(s)

THURSDAY

BREAKFAST
Chilled Fruit Juice
Buttermilk Pancakes
Soft Butter
Warm Maple Syrup
  or Honey
Beverage(s)

DINNER
Spareribs and Sauer-
  kraut
Boiled Potatoes
Rye Bread
Butter or Margarine—
  Plum Butter
Applesauce Cake
Beverage(s)

SUPPER
Cranberry Juice
Baked Lamb Patties

Baby Lima Beans
Hot Corn Muffins
Butter or Margarine—
  Syrup
Chilled Plums
Beverage(s)

FRIDAY

BREAKFAST
Orange Slices
Scrambled Eggs
Crisp Bacon
Toast
Butter or Margarine
Jelly
Beverage(s)

DINNER

V-8 Juice
Salmon Croquettes
  with Cheese
  Sauce
Buttered Green Peas
Molded Fruit Salad

Rolls, wholewheat
Butter or Margarine
Devils Food Cake
Beverage(s)

SUPPER
Cheese Souffle
Tomato Sauce

Stuffed Celery, Ripe
  Olives
Chocolate Chip
  Oatmeal Cookies
Beverage(s)

SATURDAY

BREAKFAST
  Stewed Prunes,
     Lemon Slices
  Assorted Cold Cereals
        or
  Oatmeal, with Cream
  Lemon Danish
  Butter or Margarine
  Beverage(s)

DINNER
  Swiss Steak
  Baked Potato
  Julienne Carrots
  Creamy Cole Slaw

  Rolls
  Butter or Margarine
  Chilled Pineapple Chunks
  Beverage(s)

SUPPER
  Cream of Asparagus
     Soup
  Assorted Sandwiches
  Celery Sticks, Pickles
  Cinnamon Apple Cup
     Cakes with Lemon
     Sauce
  Beverage(s)

48th Week

SUNDAY	**MONDAY**

BREAKFAST
Grapefruit and
Orange Sections
Bacon Omelet
Golden Toast
Butter or Margarine
Jam or Marmalade
Beverage(s)

BREAKFAST
Chilled Fruit Juice
Assorted Cold Cereals
or
Wheatena, with Cream
Cheese Danish Roll
Butter or Margarine
Beverage(s)

DINNER
Roast Lamb, Mint
Jelly
Mashed Potatoes
Cauliflower with
Cheese Sauce
Tossed Green Salad/
dressing
Rolls
Butter or Margarine
Frozen Peach Short-
cake/Topping
Beverage(s)

DINNER
Braised Calves Liver

Parsley Buttered
Potatoes
Breaded Tomato and
Onions
Rolls, homemade
Butter or Margarine
Banana Bread Pudding
Beverage(s)

SUPPER
Individual Beef
Pot Pie
Cottage Cheese and
Chives Salad
Rolls, homemade
Butter or Margarine
Sponge Cake
Beverage(s)

SUPPER
Split Pea Soup
Hot Roast Beef Sand-
wich with Gravy
Strawberry Gelatin with
Grapes
Chocolate Brownies

Beverage(s)

TUESDAY

BREAKFAST
  Stewed Apricots
  Fried Egg
  Hickory Smoked
    Bacon
  Golden Toast
  Butter or Margarine—
    Jam
  Beverage(s)

DINNER
  Beef Stew with
    Vegetables
  Tossed Salad,
    French dressing
  Hot Pan Rolls
  Butter or Margarine
  Fruit Cobbler—
    Nutmeg Flavored/
    Topping
  Beverage(s)

SUPPER
  Tomato Juice
  Swiss Steak
  Hashed Brown
    Potatoes
  Cabbage Salad/
    dressing
  Bread
  Butter or Margarine
  Dutch Apple Cake/
    Chocolate Frost-
    ing
  Beverage(s)

WEDNESDAY

BREAKFAST
  Chilled Pineapple Juice
  Assorted Cold Cereals
    or
  Oatmeal, with cream
  Hot Rolls
  Butter or Margarine
  Jelly
  Beverage(s)

DINNER
  Baked Southern
    Cured Ham
  Glazed Sweet Potatoes

  Buttered Green Peas
  Pear and Shredded
    Cheese Salad/
    dressing
  Hot Bran Muffins
  Butter or Margarine
  Lemon Fluff
  Beverage(s)

SUPPER
  Beef Noodle Soup
  Baked Lamb Patties

  Creole Lima Beans
  Bread
  Butter or Margarine
  Rice Bavarian/
    Maple Sauce
  Beverage(s)

THURSDAY	FRIDAY
BREAKFAST	**BREAKFAST**
Grapefruit Sections, Grenadine	Chilled Prune Juice
Poached Egg on Buttered Toast	Old Fashioned Waffles
Apple Danish Roll	Honey Butter
Butter or Margarine	Warm Maple Syrup
Beverage(s)	Beverage(s)

THURSDAY

BREAKFAST
Grapefruit Sections,
 Grenadine
Poached Egg on
 Buttered Toast
Apple Danish Roll
Butter or Margarine
Beverage(s)

DINNER
American Chop Suey
Fluffy Buttered Rice
Carrot Sticks, Pickles,
 Green and Black
 Olives
Rolls, homemade
Butter or Margarine
Maple-Nut Mold/
 Custard Sauce
Beverage(s)

SUPPER
Pineapple Juice
Sliced Pork Sandwich
Brown Gravy
Beet and Onion
 Salad
Bread
Butter or Margarine
Chilled Butterscotch
 Pudding
Beverage(s)

FRIDAY

BREAKFAST
Chilled Prune Juice
Old Fashioned Waffles
Honey Butter
Warm Maple Syrup
Beverage(s)

DINNER
Creamed Salmon
 and Peas on Hot
 Biscuits
Asparagus Salad with
 Sliced Eggs/French
 Dressing
Biscuits
Butter or Margarine—
 Apple Butter
Chilled Pears
Beverage(s)

SUPPER
Celery and Tomato
 Soup—Saltines
Spanish Omelette
Buttered Green Peas
Bread
Butter or Margarine
Homemade Applesauce
Baked Rice Pudding/
 Topping
Beverage(s)

SATURDAY

BREAKFAST
  Chilled Fresh
    Melon Slice
  Assorted Cold Cereals
    or
  Cream of Wheat,
    warm milk
  Cinnamon Nut Roll
  Butter or Margarine
  Beverage(s)

DINNER
  Spaghetti and Meat
    Sauce
  Buttered Broccoli Cuts
  Lettuce Wedges
    with Blue Cheese
    and Mayonnaise

  Sesame Rolls, homemade
  Butter or Margarine
  Spumoni (Ice Cream)
  Beverage(s)

SUPPER
  Apple Juice
  Peanut Butter and
    Bacon Sandwich
  Pear and Bing Cherry
    Salad   with
    Dressing and Ground
    Peanuts
  Whipped Fruit Gelatin/
    Topping
  Beverage(s)

49th Week

SUNDAY

BREAKFAST
Chilled Melon
Scrambled Eggs
Hickory Smoked
Bacon
Blueberry Muffin
Butter or Margarine
Beverage(s)

DINNER
Roast Pork
Glazed Sweet
Potatoes
Stewed Tomatoes

Carrot and Raisin
Salad
Rolls, homemade
Butter or Margarine
Ice Cream/Straw-
berry Sauce
Beverage(s)

SUPPER
Beef Broth
Spanish Rice (with
chopped meat)
Rolls, graham
Butter or Margarine
Blueberry Puff
Beverage(s)

MONDAY

BREAKFAST
Assorted Fruit Juices
Selected Cold Cereals
or
Oatmeal, with cream
Toast, Buttered
Jelly
Beverage(s)

DINNER
Corned Beef and
Cabbage
Boiled Potatoes
Jellied Vegetable
Salad
Rolls
Butter or Margarine
Raisin Pudding
Beverage(s)

SUPPER
Chili Con Carne
Summer Squash
Carrot Strips—Celery—
Olives
Bread, wholewheat
Butter or Margarine
Whipped Fruit Gelatin
Beverage(s)

TUESDAY	WEDNESDAY

BREAKFAST
- Orange Sections
- Poached Egg on
  Buttered Toast
- Hot Rolls
- Butter or Margarine–
  Jam
- Beverage(s)

BREAKFAST
- Bananas with Cream
- Golden French Toast
- Maple Syrup or Honey
- Canadian Bacon
- Beverage(s)

DINNER
- Baked Ham   with
  Raisin Sauce
- Mashed Sweet Potatoes
- Spinach, buttered
- Waldorf Salad
- Rolls, homemade
- Butter or Margarine
- Steamed Fig Pudding/
  Topping
- Beverage(s)

DINNER
- Beef Stroganoff
- Buttered Noodles
- Pear Salad/dressing

- Sesame Seed Rolls
- Butter or Margarine
- Cranberry and Raisin
  Pie
- Beverage(s)

SUPPER
- Corn Chowder
- Fried Vienna Sausages
- Buttered Broccoli
  Spears
- Bread, wholewheat
- Butter or Margarine
- Beet and Onion
  Salad
- Angel Food Cake/
  Frosted
- Beverage(s)

SUPPER
- Veal Cutlet
  Tomato Sauce
- Buttered Whole Leaf
  Spinach
- Vegetable Salad/
  dressing
- Brownies
- Beverage(s)

THURSDAY	FRIDAY

BREAKFAST
Assorted Juices
Selected Cold Cereal
   or
Wheatena, with cream
Corn Muffins
Butter or Margarine—
   Jelly
Beverage(s)

DINNER
Fried Chicken and
   Gravy
Mashed Potatoes
Fried Parsnips
Buttered Green
   Peas
Jellied Pineapple and
   Cucumber Salad
Bread, white and dark
Butter or Margarine
Jelly Roll (cake)

Beverage(s)

SUPPER
Beef Rice Soup
Green Peppers Stuffed
   (with ground meat
   and tomato sauce)
Carrot Sticks
Bread, white and dark
Butter or Margarine
Apple Crisp
Beverage(s)

BREAKFAST
Grapefruit Half
Fried Egg
Plantation Sausage
Toast
Butter or Margarine—
   Jam
Beverage(s)

DINNER
V-8 Juice
Shrimp Creole
Steamed Buttered
   Rice
Scalloped Egg Plant

French Bread
Butter or Margarine
Cherry Cobbler/
   Topping
Beverage(s)

SUPPER
Crispy Corn Bread
Warm Maple Syrup
Sliced American Cheese
Country Fried Potatoes

Fruit Salad /dressing

Hot Lima Beans and
   Corn
Chilled Chocolate
   Pudding
Beverage(s)

SATURDAY

BREAKFAST
Assorted Juices
Buttermilk Pancakes
Honey Butter
Warm Maple Syrup
Grilled Ham
Beverage(s)

DINNER
Beef Hash (including
potatoes)
Green Beans, buttered
Bread, white and dark
Butter or Margarine
Hot Apple Pie
Beverage(s)

SUPPER
Beef Bouillon
Chicken Chow Mein

Buttered Rice
Jellied Vegetable
Salad
Chilled Pears
Beverage(s)

50th Week

SUNDAY

BREAKFAST
  Chilled Orange Juice
  Country Fresh Egg
  Grilled Sausages
  Almond Nut Dough-
    nuts
  Butter or Margarine
  Beverage(s)

DINNER
  Roast Pork and
    Gravy
  Whipped Yams
  Lima Beans
  Cottage Cheese Salad
  Rolls
  Butter or Margarine
  Orange Chiffon Cake/
    Topping
  Beverage(s)

SUPPER
  Cream of Corn
    Soup
  Cold Cuts (including
    cheese and slice of
    Roast Pork)
  Catsup—Mustard—
    Pickles—Olives
  Bread, white and dark
  Butter or Margarine
  Oatmeal Crunch Cookies
  Beverage(s)

MONDAY

BREAKFAST
  Fruit in Season
  Old Fashioned Waffles
  Crisp Bacon
  Honey or Maple Syrup
  Soft Butter
  Beverage(s)

DINNER
  Swiss Steak
  Boiled Potatoes
  Buttered Broccoli
  Carrots and Celery
    Sticks
  Bread, white and dark
  Butter or Margarine
  Purple Plums
  Beverage(s)

SUPPER
  Potato and Onion
    Soup
  Link Sausages with
    Apple Ring
  Creamed Carrots
  Head Lettuce
    Russian Dressing
  Bread, white and dark
  Butter or Margarine
  Hermits (cookies)
  Beverage(s)

TUESDAY	WEDNESDAY

BREAKFAST
Assorted Juices
Poached Egg on
    Buttered Toast
Orange Pineapple
    Danish Roll
Butter or Margarine
Beverage(s)

BREAKFAST
Half Grapefruit
Selected Cold Cereal
    or
Cream of Wheat,
    with cream
Golden Toast
Butter or Margarine—
    Jelly
Beverage(s)

DINNER
Lamb Stew (carrots,
    peas, celery)
Graham Rolls
Butter or Margarine
Gingerale Fruit Salad/
    dressing
Filled Cookies
Beverage(s)

DINNER
Spaghetti and Meat
    Sauce
Buttered Leaf Spinach
Tossed Green Salad/
    Italian Dressing
French Bread
Butter or Margarine
Lemon Pie
Beverage(s)

SUPPER
Beef Bouillon
Spiced Ham and
    Pimiento Loaf
    Sandwiches
Stewed Tomatoes

Butter or Margarine
Creamy Tapioca
    Pudding
Beverage(s)

SUPPER
Cream of Spinach
    Soup
Eggs a la King on an
    English Muffin,
    buttered
Head Lettuce Salad

Cooked Apple Slices
    with Cinnamon
    Sauce
Beverage(s)

THURSDAY

BREAKFAST
Chilled Fruit Juice
Buttermilk Pancakes
Soft Butter
Warm Maple Syrup
or Honey
Beverage(s)

DINNER
Baked Chicken,
Gravy
Whipped Potatoes
Sliced Buttered Beets
Apple-Date-Celery
Salad/dressing
Rolls, homemade
Butter or Margarine
Individually Molded
Coffee Bavarian

Beverage(s)

SUPPER
French Onion
Soup
Spanish Rice
Orange and Green
Pepper Salad/
dressing
Hard Rolls, sesame
seed
Butter or Margarine
Chilled Apricots
Beverage(s)

FRIDAY

BREAKFAST
Orange Slices
Scrambled Eggs
Crisp Bacon
Toast
Butter or Margarine
Jelly
Beverage(s)

DINNER
Chilled Vegetable Juice
Baked Stuffed Haddock

Creamy Mashed Potatoes
Glazed Coin Sized
Carrots
Rolls, petite size
Butter or Margarine
Blueberry Pie, home
baked
Beverage(s)

SUPPER
Cream of Celery Soup
Saltines
Spanish Omelette
Tomato Aspic Salad
Chocolate Cupcakes
Beverage(s)

SATURDAY

BREAKFAST
  Stewed Prunes,
      Lemon Slices
  Assorted Cold Cereals
          or
  Oatmeal, with cream
  Plain Doughnut
  Butter or Margarine
  Beverage(s)

DINNER
  Veal Roast
  Hashed Brown
      Potatoes
  Peas and Onions
  Tomato and Cucumber
      Salad
  Baking Powder Biscuits

  Butter or Margarine—
      Plum Butter
  Coconut Frosted Cake

  Beverage(s)

SUPPER
  Ham and Sweet Potato
      Casserole
  Buttered Green Beans
  Bread, wholewheat
  Butter or Margarine
  Applesauce and
      Cookies
  Beverage(s)

51st Week

SUNDAY	MONDAY
BREAKFAST	**BREAKFAST**
Grapefruit and	Chilled Fruit Juice
Orange Sections	Assorted Cold Cereals
Bacon Omelet	or
Golden Toast	Wheatena, with cream
Butter or Margarine	Cheese Danish Roll
Jam or Marmalade	Butter or Margarine
Beverage(s)	Beverage(s)
DINNER	**DINNER**
The First Ribs—	Beef Hash
Roast of Beef	Squash, (baked
Yorkshire Pudding	with brown sugar)
Parsnips, buttered	
Creamed Carrots	Cole Slaw
Hot Parkerhouse	Buttered Brussel
Rolls	Sprouts
Butter or Margarine	Bread, white and dark
Mincemeat Pie	Butter or Margarine
Beverage(s)	Bread Pudding, with
	Honey Sauce
	Beverage(s)
SUPPER	**SUPPER**
Cream of Celery	Tomato Juice
Soup	Hot Pork Sandwich
Cold Plate—Ham,	Mashed Turnips
Beef, Cheese	Sunshine Cake
Potato Salad	Beverage(s)
Rolls, petite	
Butter or Margarine	
Baked Meringues	
with Apricot	
Sauce	
Beverage(s)	

TUESDAY

BREAKFAST
  Stewed Apricots
  Fried Egg
  Hickory Smoked
    Bacon
  Golden Toast
  Butter or Margarine—
    Jam
  Beverage(s)

DINNER
  Lamb Patties,
    Mint Jelly
  Lyonnaise Potatoes

  Buttered Cauliflower

  Tossed Salad/dressing

  Rolls, homemade
  Butter or Margarine
  Oatmeal Molasses
    Cookies
  Beverage(s)

SUPPER
  Beef Stew with
    Vegetables
  Steamed Rice
  Corn Bread
  Butter or Margarine—
    Plum Butter
  Chilled Apricots
  Beverage(s)

WEDNESDAY

BREAKFAST
  Chilled Pineapple Juice
  Assorted Cold Cereals
    or
  Oatmeal, with cream
  Hot Rolls
  Butter or Margarine—
    Jelly
  Beverage(s)

DINNER
  Grilled Calves Liver
    and Bacon
  Buttered Parsley
    Potatoes
  Stewed Whole
    Tomatoes
  Rolls
  Butter or Margarine
  Shredded Cabbage and
    Carrot Salad
  Chilled Peaches
  Beverage(s)

SUPPER
  Chicken and Rice
    Soup
  Broiled Meat Patty
  Buttered Green Beans
  Bread
  Butter or Margarine
  Whipped Fruit Gelatin
  Beverage(s)

THURSDAY	FRIDAY

BREAKFAST
    Grapefruit Sections,
      Grenadine
    Poached Egg on
      Buttered Toast
    Apple Danish Roll
    Butter or Margarine
    Beverage(s)

BREAKFAST
    Chilled Prune Juice
    Old Fashioned Waffles
    Honey Butter
    Warm Maple Syrup
    Beverage(s)

DINNER
    Pizza Pie
    Tossed Green Salad/
      dressing
    Applesauce
    Molasses Drop
      Cookies
    Beverage(s)

DINNER
    Cheese Souffle
    Green Beans,
      French Style
    Baked Potato
    Spiced Pear
    Assorted Homemade
      Cookies
    Beverage(s)

SUPPER
    Navy Bean Soup

    Turkey Salad with
      Tomato Wedges

    Rolls
    Butter or Margarine
    Devils Food Cake
      Squares/Icing
    Beverage(s)

SUPPER
    French Onion
      Soup
    Tomato Stuffed with
      Tunafish Salad
    Buttered Asparagus
    Corn Muffin, hot
    Butter or Margarine—
      Apple Butter
    Banana Cream Pie
    Beverage(s)

SATURDAY

BREAKFAST
  Chilled Fresh
     Melon Slice
  Assorted Cold Cereals
          or
  Cream of Wheat,
     warm milk
  Cinnamon Raisin
     Pecan Roll
  Butter or Margarine
  Beverage(s)

DINNER
  Chili Con Carne
  Buttered Rice
  Celery Hearts and
     Stuffed Olives
  Poppy Seed Hard
     Rolls
  Butter or Margarine
  Butterscotch Pudding
  Beverage(s)

SUPPER
  Vegetable Soup
  Chicken Pot Pie
  Pear and Cottage
     Cheese Salad
  Hot Parker House Rolls

  Butter or Margarine
  Frosted Yellow Cake
     Slice
  Beverage(s)

52nd Week

SUNDAY	MONDAY

BREAKFAST
Chilled Melon
Scrambled Eggs
Hickory Smoked
   Bacon
Sugar Doughnut
Beverage(s)

BREAKFAST
Assorted Fruit Juices
Selected Cold Cereals
   or
Oatmeal, with cream
Toast, buttered
Beverage(s)

DINNER
Pineapple Juice
Assorted Relish Tray
Baked Ham
   Raisin Sauce
Candied Sweet Potato

Buttered Green Beans,
   French Style
Home-Baked Nut Bread

Butter or Margarine
Orange Sherbet and
   Vanilla Cookies
Beverage(s)

DINNER
Veal Stroganoff
Buttered Rice
Buttered Broccoli
Perfection Salad
Bread
Butter or Margarine
Caramel Custard
Beverage(s)

SUPPER
Corn Chowder
   Saltines
Assorted Sandwiches
Mixed Green Salad/
   dressing
Pineapple Cheese Cake

Beverage(s)

SUPPER
Baked Green Peppers
   (stuffed with ground
   meat, tomato sauce)
Jellied Fruit Salad
Raisin Bread
Butter or Margarine
Fruit Cake
Beverage(s)

TUESDAY	WEDNESDAY

BREAKFAST
- Orange Sections
- Poached Egg on
  - Buttered Toast
- Hot Rolls
- Butter or Margarine—
  - Jam
- Beverage(s)

DINNER
- Lamb Stew with
  - Dumplings
- Buttered Green Peas
- Buttered Carrot Rings
- Cole Slaw
- Bread
- Butter or Margarine
- Pound Cake
- Beverage(s)

SUPPER
- Chilled Tomato Juice
- Turkey Salad
- Cranberry Sauce
- Stuffed Celery
- Rolls, sesame
- Butter or Margarine
- Mincemeat Cookies
- Beverage(s)

BREAKFAST
- Bananas with Cream
- Golden French Toast
- Maple Syrup or Honey
- Canadian Bacon
- Beverage(s)

DINNER
- Chicken and Vegetable
  - Pie
- Candied Sweet Potatoes

- Shredded Lettuce/
  - dressing
- Bread
- Butter or Margarine
- Orange Date Nut Cake
- Beverage(s)

SUPPER
- Puree Mongole
- Beef and Rice Balls
- Wax Beans, Buttered
- Jellied Fruit Salad/
  - dressing
- Rolls
- Butter or Margarine
- Crisp Molasses Cookies

- Beverage(s)

THURSDAY	FRIDAY
BREAKFAST	**BREAKFAST**
Assorted Juices	Grapefruit Half
Selected Cold Cereal	Fried Egg
or	Plantation Sausage
Wheatena, with cream	Toast
Corn Muffins	Butter or Margarine—
Butter or Margarine	Jam
Jelly	Beverage(s)
Beverage(s)	
DINNER	**DINNER**
Meat Loaf	Salmon Loaf
Boiled Potatoes	Parsley Potatoes
Buttered Cut Green	Carrot Strips
Beans	Braised Celery
Fruited Gelatin	Bread
Bread	Butter or Margarine
Butter or Margarine	Apple Crisp
Lemon Coconut Cake	Beverage(s)
Beverage(s)	
SUPPER	**SUPPER**
Navy Bean Soup	Washington Chowder,
Weiners on Rolls	Saltines
Butter—Catsup—	Creamed Eggs and
Mustard—Relish	Mushrooms on
Cole Slaw	Toast
Cottage Pudding with	Brown Sugar Crumb
Fruit Sauce	Cake with Topping
Beverage(s)	Beverage(s)

SATURDAY

BREAKFAST
  Assorted Juices
  Buttermilk Pancakes
  Honey Butter
  Warm Maple Syrup
  Grilled Ham
  Beverage(s)

DINNER
  Spanish Rice with
    Crumbled Bacon
  Shredded Cabbage and
    Apple and Nut
    Salad/dressing
  Buttered Asparagus
  Rolls
  Butter or Margarine
  Baked Honey Custard
  Beverage(s)

SUPPER
  Cream of Tomato
    Soup
  Grilled Cheese Sandwich
  Jellied Fruit Salad
  Applesauce Cake, boiled
    icing
  Beverage(s)

Extra Menu Days

"EXTRA" SUNDAY	"EXTRA" MONDAY

BREAKFAST
  Chilled Orange Juice
  Country Fresh Eggs
  Grilled Sausages
  Jelly Doughnuts
  Beverage(s)

BREAKFAST
  Fruit in Season
  Old Fashioned Waffles
  Crisp Bacon
  Honey or Maple Syrup
  Soft Butter

DINNER
  Fruit Cocktail
  Baked Chicken
    and dressing
  Mashed Potatoes
  Green Beans, buttered
  Parker House Roll
  Butter or Margarine
  Vanilla Ice Cream
    with Pineapple Sauce
    and Whipped Cream
    Rosette
  Beverage(s)

DINNER
  Baked Roast Beef Hash
    (onions and
    potatoes included in
    hash)
  Buttered Spinach
  Jellied Tomato Salad

  Bread, white and dark
  Butter or Margarine
  Lemon Refrigerator
    Dessert
  Beverage(s)

SUPPER
  Beef Broth and
    Rice
  Saltines
  Cold Plate—Ham,
    Cheese, Roast Beef
  Stuffed Celery—Olives
  Bread, wholewheat
  Butter or Margarine
  Mincemeat Fudge
    Squares
  Beverage(s)

SUPPER
  Corn Chowder
  Apple Fritters
  Hot Maple Syrup
  Chopped Raw Salad

  Chilled Queen Anne
    Cherries
  Beverage(s)

"EXTRA" TUESDAY

BREAKFAST
  Assorted Juices
  Poached Egg on
    Buttered Toast
  Apricot Danish Roll
  Butter or Margarine
  Beverage(s)

DINNER
  Liver Creole
  Mashed Potatoes
  Buttered Cauliflower
  Jellied Pineapple and
    Carrot Salad
  Bread
  Butter or Margarine
  Baked Custard
  Beverage(s)

SUPPER
  Apple Juice
  Spanish Rice
  Molded Cottage
    Cheese Salad
  Rolls
  Butter or Margarine
  Chilled Pears
  Beverage(s)

"EXTRA" WEDNESDAY

BREAKFAST
  Half Grapefruit
  Selected Cold Cereal
      or
  Cream of Wheat,
    with cream
  Golden Toast
  Butter or Margarine—
    Jelly
  Beverage(s)

DINNER
  Lamb Stew with
    Dumplings
  Buttered Peas
  Dark Bran Muffins
  Chopped Spinach
    with Bacon
  Butter or Margarine
  Golden Chiffon Cake

  Beverage(s)

SUPPER
  Cream of Celery Soup

  Corned Beef Hash
  Bread, white and dark
  Butter or Margarine
  Fruited Gelatin
  Beverage(s)

"EXTRA" THURSDAY

BREAKFAST
  Chilled Fruit Juice
  Buttermilk Pancakes
  Soft Butter
  Warm Maple Syrup
    or Honey
  Beverage(s)

DINNER
  New England Boiled
    Dinner
    (includes potatoes,
    onions, etc.)
  Buttered Peas
  Fruit Salad
  Rolls
  Butter or Margarine
  Lemon Coconut Cake
  Beverage(s)

SUPPER
  Cold Cuts (Ham,
    Beef, and Cheese)
  Bread, white and dark
  Butter or Margarine
  Green Salad
  Raspberry Jumble
    Cookies
  Beverage(s)

"EXTRA" FRIDAY

BREAKFAST
  Orange Slices
  Scrambled Eggs
  Crisp Bacon
  Toast
  Butter or Margarine–
    Jelly
  Beverage(s)

DINNER
  Fried Fish Fillets
  Parsley Buttered
    Potatoes
  Baked Tomatoes
  Waldorf Salad
  Bread
  Butter or Margarine
  Lemon-Filled Cupcake
  Beverage(s)

SUPPER
  Potato Chowder
  Tunafish and Celery
    Salad
  Potato Chips
  Pickles
  Custard Pie
  Beverage(s)

"EXTRA" SATURDAY

BREAKFAST
Stewed Prunes,
Lemon Slices
Assorted Cold Cereals
or
Oatmeal, with cream
Lemon Streusel Danish
Butter or Margarine
Beverage(s)

DINNER
Baked Ham with
Raisin sauce
Browned Potatoes
Green Beans
Jellied Pineapple and
Carrot Salad
Bread, white and dark
Butter or Margarine
Maple Nut Cake
with Topping
Beverage(s)

SUPPER
Turkey Goulash
Lettuce and Tomato
Salad
Rolls
Butter or Margarine
Cream Cheese Apricot
Turnovers
Beverage(s)

Menus for the Holidays

New Year's Day
Leap Year, February 29th
St. Patrick's Day
Easter'
July 4th
Labor Day
Thanksgiving
Christmas

NEW YEAR'S DAY

BREAKFAST
Chilled Orange Juice
Country Fresh Eggs
Grilled Sausages
Almond Nut
  Doughnuts
Butter or Margarine
Beverage(s)

DINNER
Wine
Roast Duck
  Burgundy
Glazed Sweet Potato

Buttered Asparagus
Jellied Cranberry
  Salad
Rolls, Butter or
  Margarine
Fruit Cake with
  Hard Sauce
Beverage(s)

SUPPER
Smorgasbord
Sliced Cold Turkey
  and Baked Ham
Hot Rolls, butter or
  margarine
Cranberry Sauce, un-
  strained
Cabbage, Almond,
  Marshmallow and
  Pineapple Salad
Date Nut Bread
Relishes
Fresh Fruits (a variety)
Meringue Kisses
  (sprinkled with green
  and red sugar)

Chocolate Pinwheel Cookies
Beverage(s)

IS IT LEAP YEAR?
IF SO, THIS IS FOR
FEBRUARY 29TH

BREAKFAST
  Grapefruit and Orange
    Sections
  Bacon Omelet
  Golden Toast
  Butter or Margarine
  Jam or Marmalade
  Beverage(s)

DINNER
  Pork Loin Roast,
    Gravy
  Mashed Potatoes
  Buttered Peas
  Vegetable Salad/
    Dressing
  Oatmeal Rolls
  Butter or Margarine
  Golden Chiffon Cake

  Beverage(s)

SUPPER
  Oyster Stew
  Grilled Cheese Sandwich
  Tomato Aspic
  Cornflake Kisses
  Beverage(s)

ST. PATRICK'S DAY

BREAKFAST
  Chilled Melon
  Scrambled Eggs
  Hickory Smoked
    Bacon
  Cinnamon Raisin
    Pecan Rolls
  Beverage(s)

DINNER
  Wine
  Roast Rolled Shoulder
    of Lamb, Boulangere

              or

  Corned Beef and
    Cabbage
  Rolls
  Butter or Margarine—
    Mint Jelly
  Green Gelatin and Half
    Pear Salad/dressing

  Peas, buttered
  Angel Food Cake/
    Topping (use green
    coloring)
  Beverage(s)

SUPPER
  Split Pea Soup
  Ham and Egg Salad
  Potato Salad
  Rolls
  Butter or Margarine
  Green Olives and Pickles
  Asparagus, buttered
  Ice Cream
  Beverage(s)

EASTER SUNDAY	JULY 4th

BREAKFAST
Chilled Orange Juice
Country Fresh Eggs
Grilled Sausages
Cinnamon Doughnuts

Butter or Margarine
Beverage(s)

DINNER
Lamb Roast, Pan
 Gravy
Parsleyed Buttered
 Potatoes
Creamed Asparagus
 (or buttered)
Fruit Salad
Rolls
Butter or Margarine
Golden Chiffon Cake
 with Topping
Beverage(s)

SUPPER
Cream of Celery
 Soup
Cold Plate—Lamb,
 Beef, Ham, Cheese
Bread, white and dark
Butter or Margarine
Relishes
Ice Cream
Coconut Peanut
 Butter Stick
 Cookies
Beverage(s)

BREAKFAST
Orange Juice
Selected Cold Cereals
Crisp Bacon and
 Fried Eggs
Toast
Butter or Margarine—Jam
Glazed Doughnuts
Beverage(s)

DINNER
Oven Fried Chicken
Mashed Potatoes
Green Beans
Lettuce and Tomato
 Salad/dressing
Rolls or Baking Powder
 Biscuits
Butter or Margarine
 and Honey
Strawberry Pie
Beverage(s)

SUPPER
Picnic Supper
 (outdoors)
Beer and/or Lemonade
Sliced Ham
Weiners
Weiner Rolls
Chopped Raw Slaw
German Potato Salad
Fudge Loaf Cake
Ice Cream in Cups
Beverage(s)

LABOR DAY

BREAKFAST
> Orange, Tomato
> or Prune Juice
> Soft Cooked Eggs
> Toast
> Butter or Margarine
> Dutch Apple Coffee
> Cake with Topping
> Beverage(s)

DINNER
> Wine
> Roast Turkey
> Dressing   and
> Giblet Gravy
> Browned Parsnips
> Buttered Green Beans
> Mashed Potatoes
> Stuffed Celery Sticks
> Oatmeal Rolls, Butter
> or Margarine
> Lemon Refrigerator
> Dessert
> Beverage(s)

SUPPER
> Celery Soup
> Roast Beef Sandwiches
> Potato Chips
> Orange and Grapefruit
> Salad/dressing
> Cherry Pie
> Beverage(s)

THANKSGIVING

BREAKFAST
> Chilled Melon
> Scrambled Eggs
> Hickory Smoked
> Bacon
> Toast, Buttered
> Jelly
> Beverage(s)

DINNER
> Wine
> Roast Turkey
> Dressing
> Giblet Gravy
> Buttered Parsnips
> Mashed Potatoes
> Buttered Peas
> Waldorf Salad with
> Honey Dressing
> Radishes and Olives
> and Celery
> Rolls
> Butter or Margarine
> Pumpkin Pie
> Beverage(s)

SUPPER
> Tomato Juice—Hors
> d'Oeuvres
> Assorted Cold Meats
> and Cheese
> Relish Tray including
> Pickled Pears and
> Peaches—Carrot
> and Celery Curls
> Bread, white and dark
> Butter or Margarine
> Fresh Fruit, (various
> kinds)
> Beverage(s)

CHRISTMAS

BREAKFAST
  Chilled Orange Juice
  Country Fresh Eggs
  Grilled Sausages
  Lemon-Filled Doughnuts
  Beverage(s)

DINNER
  Wine and/or Apple Juice
  Roast Turkey
      Dressing   and
      Giblet Gravy
  Whipped Potatoes
  Buttered Asparagus Spears
  Spiced Pears—Brandied
      Peaches
  Olives (green and black)—
      Celery
  Waldorf Salad
  Raisin Bread   butter
      or margarine
  Mincemeat Pie—Apple Pie
  Beverage(s)

SUPPER
  Smorgasbord
  Cranberry Juice
  Sliced Baked Ham,
      Turkey, Assorted Cheeses
  Potato Salad
  Rolls, butter or
      margarine
  Relishes
  Fresh Fruits (Grapes, etc.)
  Three Bean Salad
  Assortment of Homemade
      Christmas Cookies
  Ice Cream Cups
  Beverage(s)

Special Menus and Diets for the Sick

The regular diet is used for persons who require no dietary restrictions. It is planned to meet all the requirements as established by the Food and Nutrition Board of the National Research Council, and to stimulate good food habits. The regular diet should include all the basic seven foods.

MILK: Two or more glasses daily for adults.
VEGETABLES: Two or more servings daily besides potato.
FRUITS: Two or more servings daily.
EGGS: Three to five a week, one daily preferred.
MEAT, CHEESE, FISH, FOWL: One or more servings daily.
CEREAL AND BREAD: Two or more servings daily.
BUTTER: Two or more tablespoons daily.

The Calorie Restricted or the Reducing Diet

The low calorie diet is a modification of the normal diet pattern in that the prescribed allowance has a caloric value below the total energy requirement for the day. The level of caloric intake prescribed for a moderate reduction program may range between 1,000 and 1,500 calories for women and between 1,500 and 2,000 calories for men. Excessive weight is due to the taking into the system of more food than it can use in daily living. This does not imply that one is eating exceptional quantities of food. It is merely a case of one's eating more than one needs of certain energy-producing foods.

Many unpleasant and sometimes fatal illnesses are associated with obesity. Some of these are: diabetes, heart disease, kidney disturbances, gall bladder trouble, backaches and sore feet.

The changing of food habits is a most important adjustment for a person to accept and learn to do. Changing easygoing ways is not easy, especially when one must relinquish sweets, rich gravies, and quantities of bread, etc., but a person can—if he or she honestly tries. The dieter should not become discouraged, however. Psychologists tell us that we expect far too much of ourselves, and when we fall short of our demands on ourselves we grow tense and discontented. The main purpose of a diet is not to try to prove to the world that the dieter is super-human. The person on a diet should be willing to accept a momentary lapse as an understandably human error—and keep trying!

By properly appraising height and the size of frame, the person wishing to diet can estimate how many pounds he (or she) must lose in order to arrive at the weight that is best.

SPECIAL DIET MENUS

Approx. 601 Calories
Steaming Bouillon—1 cup
Juicy Roast Leg of Lamb—
   4 oz.
Fresh Green Peas—½ cup
Cauliflower—½ cup
Tomato Aspic on Lettuce
   Leaf—½ cup
Rye Wafer (2)—Pat of
   Butter
Old Fashioned Ginger-
   bread—one small
   portion
Black Coffee

Approx. 608 Calories
Hot or Cold Consomme—
   1 cup
Sizzling Broiled Steak—
   3 oz., boneless
Broiled Mushroom Caps—
   2 large
Green Beans—½ cup
Crisp Garden Salad—½ cup
Lemon Juice Dressing—
   1 tbsp.
Sliced American Cheese—
   1 slice

Approx. 372 Calories
Shrimp Salad Supreme—
   8 shrimp
Lettuce Salad, Dressing
Rye Wafer
Fluffy Prune Whip—¾ cup
Skim Milk or Black Coffee

Approx. 588 Calories
Chilled Tomato Juice—½ cup
Broiled Halibut Steak,
   Lemon Wedge—4 oz.
Broccoli Spears—1 stalk,
   5 in. long
Fresh Steamed Carrots—
   ½ cup
Cottage Cheese Salad
   with Chives—½ cup
Apricot Halves—Vanilla
   Wafer—4 halves, one
   cookie
Black Coffee

Approx. 386 Calories
Chilled Chicken Slices—
   3½ oz.
Low Calorie Dressing—1 tsp.
Hot Asparagus—4 med. stalks
Fresh Tomato Wedges—medium
Enriched Bread—1 slice
Cluster of Fresh Grapes
   (Tokay 20)
Skim Milk or Black Coffee

Approx. 455 Calories
Hearty Vegetable Soup—1 cup
Chopped Lean Beef Patty—
   4 oz.
Rosy Onion Rings—3
Savory Green Beans—2/3 cup
Chilled Cantaloupe—½
Skim Milk or Black Coffee—
   1 cup

The dieter should not be impatient or try to go too fast. A weight loss of 1½ pounds a week, or approximately 5 pounds a month, is as rapid as is usually advisable.

If this seems slow, it is well to remember that a gradual reduction of 5 pounds a month will, in a year, account for 60 unwanted pounds.

CALORIE CHART

Dairy Foods	Size of Portion	Calories
Milk, whole	1 glass (8 oz.)	170
Milk, skim or buttermilk	1 glass (8 oz.)	85
Milk, chocolate drink	1 glass (8 oz.)	185
Cheese, American or Swiss	1 in. cube or med. slice (1 oz.)	110
Cheese foods, Cheddar-type	2 tablespoons (1 oz.)	90
Cheese, Cottage, creamed	2 tablespoons (1 oz.)	30
Cheese, Cream	2x1x½ in. or 2 tbsp.	110
Butter	1 tablespoon (½ oz.)	100
Butter	teaspoon or small pat	35
Cream, light style	2 tablespoons	60
Cream, heavy, whipped	1 heaping tablespoon	50
Half-and-half	¼ cup	80
Ice cream, vanilla	¼ pint (½ cup)	150
Ice cream, as for a la mode	Medium scoop (1/5 pt.)	125
Sherbet	½ cup	120

Meat, Fish, Poultry, Eggs, Legumes

Meat, Fish, Poultry, lean to medium fat, averaged	1 serving (3 oz. cooked, weight without bones)	230
Liver	1 serving (3 oz. cooked)	180
Frankfurter	1 medium (1¾ oz.)	125
Luncheon Meat	2 medium slices (2 oz.)	165
Ham, boiled or baked	1 thin slice, 5x4 in.(1 oz.)	85
Tuna or Salmon, canned	1/3 cup (2 oz.)	105
Chicken, creamed	½ cup	210
Sausage, cooked	1 link, 3 in. long (2/3 oz.)	95
Bacon, crisp	2 long slices (½ oz.)	100
Eggs	1 medium	75
Eggs, scrambled	1 egg, tbsp. milk, tsp. butter	120
Dried Beans, split peas	¾ cup, cooked	150
Baked Beans with pork	¾ cup	245
Nuts, shelled, roasted	3 tbsp. chopped 30 peanuts	150

Other Popular Main Dishes

Meat and Vegetable Stew	¾ cup	190
Cheese Fondue	Med.serving, 1½x2x2½ in.	150
Macaroni and Cheese	¾ cup	350
Spaghetti, Italian style	Large serving with cheese	420
Chicken Pie, peas, potatoes	1 pie, 3¾ in. diameter	460
Soup, Navy Bean	1 cup	190
Soup, creamed style	1 cup	200

Fruits

FRESH,UNSWEETENED	1 med. serving, average	50-100
Citrus fruit	small orange, ½ grapefruit	50
Melon	½ medium cantaloupe	50
Peach	1 medium	50
Strawberries	1 cup	55
Grapes	small bunch	55
Blackberries, Raspberries	1 cup	75
Apple, Banana, Pear	1 medium	85
Avocado	¼ medium	140
COOKED, LIGHTLY SWEETENED	½ cup	100
Apple, baked, sweetened	1 large	210
Rhubarb sauce, sweetened	½ cup	190
DRIED	¼ cup raisins, or 4 large prunes or 2 small figs, or 3-4 dates	90
Fruit Juice	½ cup	50
Tomato Juice	½ cup	25

Vegetables and Salads

Green Beans	½ cup, cooked	15
Green leafy vegetables	½ cup, cooked	25
Carrots	½ cup, cooked	20
Root, others, as Beets, Onions	½ cup, cooked	35
Squash, winter	½ cup, cooked	50
Legumes; Green Peas	½ cup, cooked	65
Baby Lima Beans	½ cup, cooked	75
Starchy, as Corn	½ cup, cooked	70
Potatoes, white	1 small potato, cooked	80
Potatoes, mashed, french fried	½ cup or 6 med. pieces	120

Vegetables and Salads (cont.)	Size of Portion	Calories
Potatoes, sweet	½ med. potato, cooked	90
Raw Carrot, Tomato	1 small to medium	25
Lettuce	¼ medium head	10
Tossed Salad, Mixed Veg.	¾ cup, without dressing	30
Coleslaw	½ cup	50
Waldorf Salad	3 heap. tablespoons	140
Potato Salad	½ cup	185
Chicken and Celery Salad	3 heap. tablespoons	185

Breadstuffs and Cereals

Bread, whole-grain or enriched	1 medium slice (¾ oz.)	60
Bread, raisin, enriched	1 medium slice (¾ oz.)	65
Cereal, cooked, whole-grain or enriched	½ cup	70
Cereal, ready-to-eat, whole-grain or enriched	½ cup	50
Corn Grits, enriched	½ cup, cooked	60
Rice or Spaghetti	½ cup, cooked	105
Noodles	½ cup, cooked	55
Biscuit	1 small (1 oz.)	95
Corn Meal Muffin	1 med., 2¾ in. dia.	105
Rolls, plain, enriched	1 small (1 oz.)	85
Rolls, sweet	1 med. (2 oz.)	180
Waffle	1 med., 4½x5½x½ in.	215
Pancake	1 thin, 4 in. diameter	60
Crackers, plain or graham	2 medium	50
Rye Wafers	2 small	45
Gingerbread	1 piece, 2 in. square	180

Pastries and Puddings

Cookies, plain	2 small or 1 large	100
Cookies, oatmeal	2 small or 1 large	115
Wafers, as vanilla	2 small, thin	45
Cupcake, not iced	1 med. 1¾ in. dia.	80
Cupcake, iced	1 med., 1¾ in. dia.	130
Brownies	1 piece, 2x2x¾ in.	140
Cake, not iced	Med. piece, 2x3x1½ in.	175-300
Cake, layer, plain icing	Med. piece, 1/6 of 6-in. cake	250-400
Cake, angel food or sponge	Small piece, 2 in. sector	115
Doughnut	1 medium	135
Eclair, chocolate	1 average	250
Pie, fruit	1/7 med.-size pie	300-350

Pastries and Puddings (cont.)	**Size of Portion**	**Calories**
Pie, custard type	1/7 med.-size pie	250-300
Pudding, cornstarch, vanilla	½ cup	140
Pudding, rice with raisins	½ cup	165
Fruit Betty	½ cup	170
Prune Whip	½ cup	100
Custard	½ cup	140
Gelatin dessert with fruit	½ cup	85
Gingerbread	1 piece, 2 in. square	180

Sauces

Cream Sauce or Milk Gravy	2 tablespoons, med. thick	50
Cheese Sauce	2 tablespoons, med. thick	65
Hollandaise Sauce	1 tablespoon	90
Catsup, Chili, Tomato Sauce	1 tablespoon	20
Custard Sauce	2 tablespoons	40
Fruit Sauce	2 tablespoons	90
Chocolate Sauce	2 tablespoons	90
Hard Sauce	2 tablespoons	100
Butterscotch Sauce	2 tablespoons	200

Candy

Candy bar, milk chocolate	1 small bar (7/8 oz.)	125
Fondant mints or patties	1 average (40 to lb.)	40
Chocolate creams	1 average (35 to lb.)	50
Fudge, plain	1 piece, 1 in. square	100
Peanut Brittle	1 piece, 2½x2½x¼ in.	120
Gumdrops	1 large or 8 small	35
Marshmallows	1 average (60 to lb.)	25

Fountain Specialties

Milk Shake, chocolate	Fountain size (5 oz. milk, 2 small scoops ice cream, 2 tablespoons syrup)	400
Malted Milk Shake	Fountain size	500
Cocoa, all milk	1 table-size (6 oz. milk)	180
Sundaes	1 medium, 2 tbsp. topping	225-335
Sodas	Fountain Size	260
Eggnog	1 large glass (8 oz. milk)	290
Carbonated drinks	1 large glass (8 oz.)	110

Fountain Specialties (cont.)

Fountain Specialties (cont.)	Size of Portion	Calories
Lemonade, slightly sweetened	1 large glass (10 oz.)	100
Ginger Ale	1 large glass (8 oz.)	80
Gingerflip	1 large glass (milk, gingerale, ice cream)	225
Mambo Shake	1 large glass (milk, banana, ice cream, lemon juice, sugar)	300
Mint Cow	1 large glass (milk, chocolate syrup, mint extract, ice cream)	320

Other Snacks

	Size of Portion	Calories
Pizza, quickly made type	1 med. serving 4-in. dia.	185
Hamburger, including bun	1 medium, lightly buttered bun	360
Hot Dog, including bun	1 medium	210
Potato Chips	10 med. or 7 large	110
Pickles	1 large dill or sweet pickle, or 4 slices cucumber pickle, or 1 tablespoon relish	15
Olives, green	2 med. olives	15
Pretzels	5 small sticks	20
Popcorn, lightly buttered	½ cup	75

Count These Too

	Size of Portion	Calories
Salad Dressing, cooked type	1 tablespoon	30
French dressing	1 tablespoon	60
mayonnaise	1 tablespoon	90
lemon juice or vinegar	1 tablespoon	3
Salad Oil	1 tablespoon	125
Jam, syrup, sugar	1 tablespoon	55

The Soft Diet

This diet represents the usual dietary step between the general liquid and regular diet. The soft diet is made up of simple, easily digested foods and contains no harsh fiber, no rich or highly seasoned foods. It is as adequate nutritionally as a normal diet.

A person on a soft diet may select foods from the regular or normal menu which offers a choice of all foods. This diet permits those foods which are mild in texture and consistency but are non-irritating to chew and digest.

SAMPLE MENU FOR THE SOFT DIET

BREAKFAST
Chilled California Grapefruit Juice
Hot Oatmeal with Cream
Scrambled Eggs
Buttered Toast with Jelly
Homogenized Milk
Coffee with Sugar and Cream

DINNER
Chilled Tomato Juice
Pot Roast of Beef
Creamy Mashed Potatoes
Buttered Carrots
Enriched Bread with Butter
Vanilla Ice Cream Slice
Homogenized Milk

SUPPER
Cream of Spinach Soup
Buttered Waxed Beans
Whipped Orange Gelatin
Tea, Sugar, Lemon

Diabetic Diets

The diabetic diet is individualized for each patient and so planned that it is physiologically correct. The physician calculates the prescription basing his allowances on:

1. The history of both the patient and his family.
2. Sex, age, weight, height and activity of the patient.
3. Type of diabetes—mild or severe.
4. Type of insulin, amount and when administered.
5. Nutritional requirements as based on the above data.

The right kind of food—in the right amount—at the right times is a most important rule for the diabetic.

Diabetes can be controlled by diet in some cases, or by diet plus insulin in others. Everyone has some sugar in his blood, but the person with diabetes has too much sugar in his blood. The diabetic does not make sufficient insulin to use the sugar from the food he eats. Almost every food he eats makes some sugar in the body. This food must be balanced with the insulin his body makes, or his doctor prescribes. Even the temporary or continued use of insulin does not mean that the diabetic can avoid constant attention to the proper diet.

Sodium Restricted Diets

The sodium restricted diet is a modification of the normal diet except that the sodium content has been restricted to a prescribed level. Other nutrients remain as nearly as possible on a level satisfactory for nutritive efficiency. Restriction of sodium is indicated for treatment of diseases in which there is edema, such as cardiac diseases, kidney disease and hypertension. There are three levels of sodium restriction: mild, moderate and severe. A number of the so-called "strongly flavored vegetables" have been included in the planning of low sodium diets. Many persons can and do eat some or all of these vegetables without distress. Consequently, the person may choose any vegetable that he feels he is able to tolerate.

Low Sodium Diet—Mild Restriction

This diet is a modification of the regular diet. A salt substitute is served instead of table salt. With this diet, you should avoid: salt at table; salt preserved foods such as ham, bacon, dried beef, salted fish, olives, bologna or sausage, anchovies, sauerkraut, bouillon cubes and meat extracts; highly salted foods such as salted nuts, potato chips, crackers, relishes, such as catsup, pickles and prepared mustards, Worcestershire or meat sauces, celery salt, garlic salt, cheese unless specially prepared without salt, peanut butter unless specially prepared without salt.

SAMPLE MENU

BREAKFAST
Chilled Florida Orange Juice
Hot Oatmeal with Cream
Scrambled Eggs
Buttered Toast with Jelly
Coffee, Sugar, Cream

LUNCHEON
Chilled Tomato Juice
Pot Roast of Beef
Fluffy Mashed Potatoes
Buttered Sliced Carrots
Lettuce Wedge
Hot Parker House Rolls
    with Butter
Homogenized Milk

DINNER
Chicken Noodle
    Casserole
Buttered Green Beans
Sliced Tomatoes
Enriched Bread with
    Butter
Sliced Peaches
Milk, Tea with Sugar
    and Lemon

Low Sodium Diet—Moderate Restrictions

On this diet you should avoid: salt in any kind of cooking and all foods listed under Mild Restriction diet; canned vegetables, meat, fish or soups unless prepared without salt; frozen peas, lima beans, frozen fish fillet; foods prepared with benzoate of soda; shellfish, except oysters; salted fat, such as butter, margarine and bacon fat; ordinary bread; anything cooked with soda, baking powder, prepared flour mixes or prepared flour; instant coffee, instant tea and postum.

Foods allowed daily under this diet are:
1. Milk; fresh, canned or powdered, 1 pint.
2. Cheese; washed cottage cheese or low Na. cheese.
3. Meat; unsalted meat, fish or fowl, 4 to 6 oz. daily.
4. Eggs; 1 or 2 daily.
5. Vegetables; any kind, fresh canned or frozen without salt.
6. Fruits; any kind.
7. Bread or alternate; low sodium bread, potatoes, puffed rice, puffed wheat, macaroni, spaghetti, noodles, any unsalted cooked cereal.
8. Fats; unsalted butter, vegetable shortenings, corn oil, lard, olive oil.
9. Dessert: pudding made with low Na. milk or part of milk allowance. Sweets: Jams, jellies, sugar, honey and hard candy.
10. Beverages; coffee, tea, cocoa (except Dutch process).

SAMPLE MENU

BREAKFAST
Chilled Florida Orange Juice
Hot Salt-Free Oatmeal
Poached Egg on Salt-Free
 Toast
Coffee, Sugar, Cream

LUNCHEON
Chilled Salt-Free
 Tomato Juice
S.F.* Pot Poast of Beef
Fluffy S.F.* Mashed Potatoes
Buttered S.F.* Sliced Carrots
Lettuce Salad with S.F.*
 Salad Dressing
Homogenized Milk

DINNER
S.F.* Chicken Noodle
 Casserole
S.F.* Buttered Green
 Beans
Sliced Tomato S.F.*
 Dressing
S.F.* Bread with Butter
Chilled Sliced Peaches
Homogenized Milk
Tea—Sugar, Lemon

S.F.*—Salt Free

Low Sodium Diet—Severe Restriction

Foods to be avoided on this diet are: All foods listed on diet No. 2 plus: Beets, beetgreens, kale, spinach, celery, chard, dandelion greens, mustard, split peas; Instant tea and coffee unless they are the 100% pure product; Milk, except dialized or low Na. milk; Dutch process cocoa, malted milk, Ovaltine.

Foods allowed daily are:
1. Milk; low Na. milk (lonalac).
2. Meat or alternate: unsalted meat, fish or fowl 4 oz. daily.
3. Eggs: one a day only.
4. Bread: low Na. bread, potato, cooked cereals, rice, spaghetti, macaroni, noodles, puffed wheat, puffed rice, shredded wheat.
5. Vegetables: use fresh or canned or frozen without salt, asparagus, beans, brussel sprouts, cabbage, squash, corn, eggplant, carrots, lettuce, peas, radishes, onions, cucumbers, tomatoes, turnips, potatoes; omit frozen lima beans and peas.
6. Fruit, any kind.
7. Fat: unsalted butter, lard, salt-free cooking fats, home-made salt-free salad dressing.
8. Desserts and sweets: sugar, honey, jam, jellies, plain gelatin, puddings made with cornstarch and low Na. milk, unsalted nuts, hard sugar candies, low sodium cookies and cakes.
9. Beverages: water, tea and coffee, low Na. milk and cocoa except Dutch process.

SAMPLE MENU
BREAKFAST

Chilled Florida Orange Juice	S.F.* Toast
S.F.* Hot Oatmeal	S.F.* Butter
Scrambled Eggs	Coffee—Sugar, Cream

LUNCHEON	SUPPER
Chilled S.F.* Tomato Juice	S.F.* Chicken and Noodle
S.F.* Pot Roast of Beef	Casserole
Creamy S.F.* Mashed	S.F.* Green Beans
Potatoes	Sliced Tomatoes, S.F.*
Buttered S.F.* Carrots	Dressing
Lettuce Salad, S.F.*	S.F.* Hot Rolls with Butter
Salad Dressing	Chilled Sliced Fruit
S.F.* Bread and Butter	Homogenized Milk, Tea—
Homogenized Milk	Sugar, Lemon
*Salt-Free	

Recipe Favorites for Low Sodium Diets

LEMON POACHED FISH

Yield: 4 portions

Ingredients

Fresh Halibut (or fresh Cod, fresh Salmon, fresh Perch, fresh Bass), sliced	1 lb.
Fresh Lemon Juice	1 tbsp.

Method

1. Cut fish into individual sized servings. Put enough water in a pan to barely cover fish, add lemon juice and bring to a boil.

2. Place the fish in the water, cover and cook below boiling point for 8 to 10 minutes.

3. Carefully remove fish from water and serve immediately with Thrifty Hollandaise Sauce.

THRIFTY HOLLANDAISE SAUCE

Yield: Approx. 1¼ cups sauce

Ingredients

Sweet Butter	2 tbsp.
Flour	2 tbsp.
Milk	1 cup
Black Pepper	1/8 tsp.
Egg Yolks, slightly beaten	2
Sweet Butter, melted	2 tbsp.
Fresh Lemon Juice	3 tbsp.

Method

1. Melt 2 tbsp. butter over low heat. Blend in flour and cook, stirring constantly, until mixture is smooth and bubbly. Remove from heat. Add milk and mix thoroughly. Return to heat, beat in pepper and 2 egg yolks. Gradually beat in melted butter and lemon juice. Serve at once.

LEMON BAKED CHICKEN

Yield: 4 to 6 portions

Ingredients

Salad Oil	¼ cup
Fresh Lemon Juice	¼ cup
Garlic, crushed	1 clove
Medium Fryer (about 3 lb.) cut into individual serving pieces	1

Method

1. Thoroughly mix salad oil, lemon juice, and garlic. Arrange chicken in a casserole and brush each piece thoroughly with lemon-oil mixture.

2. Uncover casserole for last 20 minutes to allow chicken to brown. Chicken may be kept covered for full baking time, then browned under broiler.

3. Baste again with lemon-oil mixture before broiling. Sprinkle with chopped parsley and paprika.

TOMATO SALAD SOLO

Yield: 4 portions

Ingredients

Sugar	¼ cup
Fresh Lemon Juice	¼ cup
Tomatoes, medium, sliced	3 to 4

Method

1. Mix together sugar and lemon juice. Pour over tomato slices. Chill.

2. Serve on lettuce.

CUCUMBER HERB SALAD

Yield: 4 portions

Ingredients

Fresh Lemon Juice	¼ cup
Sugar	1 tbsp.
Grated Onion	½ tsp.
Marjoram or Thyme	1/8 tsp.
Cucumber, large	1

Method

1. Mix together lemon juice, sugar, onion and marjoram or thyme. Peel cucumber, if desired; slice and marinate in lemon mixture. Chill.

2. Serve with marinade, or drain and arrange on lettuce leaves. Good, also as a garnish for meats and salads.

BROILED BEEF PATTIES

Yield: 6 portions
Ingredients

Low-Sodium Bread Crumbs	¼ cup
Fresh Lemon Juice	2 tbsp.
Onion, small, finely chopped	1
Black Pepper	¼ tsp.
Ground Beef	1 lb.
Sweet Butter	Approx. 2 tbsp.

Method

1. Moisten low-sodium bread crumbs with lemon juice. Add crumbs, onion and pepper to ground beef and mix well.

2. Form into patties and brush with sweet butter before placing under broiler. Broil approx. 5 to 6 minutes.

3. Turn, brush with sweet butter and broil until done. Makes about 6 medium-sized patties.

BREAD

Yield: 2 loaves
Ingredients

Water	2 cups
Sugar	1 tsp.
Lard	1 tsp.
Dried Yeast	1½ pkg.
Lukewarm Water	½ cup
Sifted Flour	4-6 cups

Method

Put sugar, salt and fat into a bowl. Add boiling water and cool to lukewarm. Add yeast which has been dissolved in ½ cup lukewarm water.

Add about three cups of flour; stir free from lumps and beat well. Add flour to make stiff enough to handle. Turn out on a floured board and knead until soft, smooth and elastic. This thoroughly mixes the ingredients.

Put back into a bowl; moisten top; cover and let rise in a warm place until double in bulk. Knead again.

Shape into loaves and place in baking loaf tins. Cover and let rise until double its bulk.

Then bake in a moderate oven one hour. Too hot oven causes crusts to brown too quickly before the heat has reached the center and prevents further rising.

LEMON CAKE TOP PUDDING

Yield: 8 portions
Ingredients

Sweet Butter	3 tbsp.
Sugar	1 cup
Egg Yolks	4
Flour	3 tbsp.
Fresh Lemon Juice	1/3 cup
Lemon Peel, grated	2 tsp.
Milk	1 cup
Egg Whites	4

Method

1. Cream butter, add sugar gradually and cream together until light and fluffy. Add egg yolks and beat well.

2. Add flour, lemon juice, peel; mix well. Stir in milk.

3. Beat egg whites until stiff, fold into mixture. Pour into loaf baking dish, 9 by 5 in. Set in pan of hot water and bake in a slow oven (325°F.) 40 minutes.

4. Turn thermostat to 350°F. and bake about 10 minutes or until brown. Serve either warm or chilled.

LEMON NUT COOKIES

Yield: 2 doz.
Ingredients

Unsalted Vegetable Shortening	½ cup
Sugar	¼ cup
Egg Yolk, beaten	1
Vanilla	1 tsp.
Egg White	1
Fresh Lemon Juice	2 tbsp.
Lemon Peel, grated	2 tsp.
Orange Peel, grated	2 tsp.
Sifted Flour	1¼ cups
Chopped Nuts (unsalted)	½ cup

Method

1. Cream shortening and sugar until light and fluffy.

2. Add egg yolk, vanilla, lemon juice and grated peel. Mix well.

3. Add flour, mix thoroughly. Chill one hour.

4. In a flat dish, beat egg white slightly with a fork. Dip one side of a teaspoonful of dough in egg white, then in nuts.

5. Place nut side up, about 2 in. apart on greased cooky sheet.

6. Bake at 325°F. 20 to 25 min. until lightly browned.

High Carbohydrate, High Protein, Low Fat Diets

This diet is a modification of the normal diet with all other nutrients at a level suitable for nutritive efficiency but with fat content restricted. It contains easily digested foods and omits those high in roughage or which tend to cause distress. Because of the limitation on fat content, other foods high in vitamin A are served frequently. This diet is used for conditions in which impairment of an organ associated with fat digestion is involved, such as gall bladder diseases and some liver diseases where there is impairment of the flow of bile.

Foods allowed on this diet are:

Cereals, all cooked or prepared

Breads, whole wheat or enriched white (toasted or plain), crackers

Fruits, fresh, canned, dried or frozen, fruit juices

Vegetables, potatoes, boiled, baked or mashed, all others fresh, canned or frozen except the so-called "gas forming vegetables," cooked without butter or other fat

Meat, fish, poultry, lean beef, veal, lamb, chicken livers, non-fatty fish, roasted, boiled or broiled, but not fried

Milk, skimmed milk as desired

Cheese, farmer, pot or cottage cheese

Dessert, sherbet, ices, gelatin, angel food cake, fruit, fresh, canned or frozen

Beverages, tea, coffee, fruit juices

Sweets, sugar, honey, jams, jellies

Foods limited on this diet are:

Whole milk, 1 pt. daily; Eggs, one daily; Butter or Margarine, 3 tsp. a day

All fried foods

Pies, pastry, cake (except angel food)

Nuts, peanut butter, olives, avocados, potato chips

All meats high in fat, such as pork, ham, sausage, bologna, frankfurters and bacon, goose, duck, all fatty fish or fish canned in oil

Gravies and rich sauces

Salad dressings and salad oils

Pickles, spiced or highly seasoned foods, such as horse-radish, dried beans, cucumbers, peppers, corn, unless their use causes no digestive discomfort

Bland Diet

This diet is used with much success in treating gastric disorders. Bland, as the term signifies, refers to the soothing, mildly-flavored foods that are easily handled by the digestive system. Such foods have the least tendency to cause further harm to an already damaged area in the stomach or intestines.

Foods allowed on this diet are:
Beverages: milk and milk drinks, tea, coffee, coffee substitute at the physician's discretion, not more than 1 cup a day.
Breads: rye bread without seeds, day-old white bread; melba toast; rusks; soda or oyster crackers; zwieback.
Cereal foods, refined and strained: cornflakes; cornmeal; farina; hominy grits; macaroni; noodles; pablum; puffed rice; rice; rice flakes; spaghetti; strained oatmeal, or whole wheat cereal.
Cheese: cream; cottage; mild cheddar when used in sauce.
Desserts: angel cake; sponge cake; arrowroot or sugar cookies; vanilla wafers; custard, plain ice cream; plain gelatin; junket; lady fingers; rice, bread, cornstarch or tapioca pudding; fruit whip.
Eggs; any way except fried.

Foods to avoid on this diet are:
Beverages: alcohol; soft drinks; tea and coffee except as indicated.
Breads: fresh bread and biscuits; wholegrain bread; graham crackers; pretzels; salted crackers; sweet rolls.
Cereals: bran, wholegrain cereals unless strained.
Cheese: strongly flavored.
Dessert: any containing fruit, nuts, or spices; doughnuts; gingerbread, pastries; pies, spice cake; tarts.
Egg, fried.

Foods easily digested are:
Meat: any tender or well-cooked, but not overcooked, meat, with the possible exception of pork. (Cooked by any method except frying.)

Bacon: broiled.
Vegetables: cooked vegetables.
Macaroni and Spaghetti: boiled or with cream sauce.
Bread: day old, or crisp toast.
Crackers
Milk or malted milk.
Butter, cream, olive oil.
Eggs: soft cooked by any method but frying.
Cereals.
Soups: bouillon, consomme, cream soups.
Fruit: stewed or canned. Fresh fruit; well chewed.
Puddings: custard, tapioca, gelatin, rice.
Cake: Plain, e. g. sponge, angel.
Cheese: cream, cottage cheese, ricotta.

Liquid Diets

FULL LIQUID DIET
The full liquid diet is made up of liquid foods and can include any food which becomes liquid at body temperature.

Foods allowed:
    carbonated beverage, cereal beverage, tea, cocoa, coffee in moderation
    refined or strained cooked cereals, farina, cream of rice cream of wheat, strained oatmeal
    strained cream soups, broth, bouillion, consomme
    plain ice cream, junket, gelatin, custard, sherbet, gelatin desserts
    milk and milk beverages
    eggnogs
    strained fruit juices
    pureed vegetables in soups
    hard candy, sugar, honey
    seasonings—salt, pepper, vanilla flavor, nutmeg in moderation

SAMPLE MENU—FULL LIQUID DIET

BREAKFAST	DINNER	SUPPER
Apple Juice	Cream of Tomato	Cream of Mushroom
Cream of Wheat	Soup	Soup
Cream	Pineapple Juice	Strained Orange
Tea	Baked Custard	Juice
	Milk	Junket
	Tea	Milk
		Tea

To Increase Protein Content: Use commercial protein supplement formulas or add gelatin to beverages.

To Decrease Fat Content: Omit butter, cream and margarine. Use skim milk. Limit eggs to one a day.

To Decrease Sodium Content: Omit salt in cooking. Use foods which have been processed and cooked without salt. Limit milk to one quart a day.

CLEAR LIQUID DIET

The clear liquid diet is made up of fluids which have little or no caloric value. It is used for patients post-operatively and in acute stages of many illnesses.

Foods allowed:
    carbonated beverages
    cereal beverages
    tea, coffee
    decaffeinated coffee
    plain gelatin
    clear fruit juices, strained fruit juices
    bouillion, broth, consomme
    sugar, honey, hard candy

SAMPLE MENU—CLEAR LIQUID DIET

BREAKFAST	DINNER	SUPPER
Apple Juice	Broth	Consomme
Tea	Gelatin	Gelatin
	Strained Pineapple Juice	Strained Grapefruit Juice
	Tea	Tea

Post Operative Fluids: Clear liquids are prescribed—fruit juices are omitted.

Low Sodium Diet Fluids: All broths and consommes are prepared without salt. Gelatin desserts are homemade. Commercial gelatin contains a sodium preservative.

Special Allergy Diets

The person with an allergy condition should receive medical guidance from his doctor and based on medical recommendations, a proper diet can be worked out. It is hoped that the information that follows will offer assistance in meal planning for those allergic to one or more of the staple foods: milk, eggs and wheat. Read the label carefully before using any type of prepared mix in order to determine if the product contains ingredients to be avoided on the allergy diet.

Flours

Standard recipes containing wheat flour may be altered to permit the use of other flours as follows:

Substitutes for 1 cup wheat flour: ½ cup barley flour; 1 cup corn flour; ¾ cup cornmeal (coarse); 1 scant cup cornmeal (fine); 5/8 cup potato flour; 7/8 cup rice flour; 1¼ cups rye flour; 1 cup rye meal; 1-1/3 cups ground rolled oats.

Combinations of flour to be substituted for 1 cup wheat flour:
   (1) rye flour—½ cup; potato flour—½ cup
   (2) rye flour—2/3 cup; potato flour—1/3 cup
   (3) rice flour—5/8 cup (10 tbsp.); rye flour—1/3 cup
   (4) soy flour—1 cup; potato starch flour—¾ cup

Products made with rice flour and cornmeal have rather grainy textures. In order to obtain a smoother texture, the rice flour may be mixed with liquid called for in the recipe, brought to a boil and then cooled before adding to other ingredients, or the cornmeal may be cooked.

Soy flour cannot be used as the only flour; it must be combined with another flour. A combination of flours should be thoroughly mixed with other dry ingredients.

Baked products made with flour other than wheat require long and slow baking, particularly when made without milk and eggs. Wheat flour should be sifted before measuring.

Coarse meals and flours require more leavening than wheat flour and 2½ tsp. of baking powder are recommended for each cup of coarse flour.

Batters of flours other than wheat often appear thicker or thinner than wheat flour batters.

Muffins and biscuits made of flours other than wheat often have a better texture when made in small sizes.

Cakes made with flours other than wheat are apt to be dry. Frosting and storing in a closed container tend to preserve their moisture.

Dry cereals such as rice flakes or corn flakes when crushed make an excellent breading for fowl, chops, or fish and meat patties.

Fat

Fat is the general term used in these recipes to indicate any cooking or table fat, liquid or solid. Fat, either vegetable or animal, may be used unless a particular flavor is desired.

Margarines and soy butter contain a small percentage of milk. Hydrogenated milk-free fat is available. Persons sensitive to milk can frequently tolerate butter.

Milk

Persons sensitive to cow's milk can often tolerate it in dried or evaporated form, or use milk other than cow's milk (examples: goat's milk, soy milk). It is wise to try these before eliminating milk from the diet.

Eggs

Baking powder should be increased 1 tsp. for each egg eliminated in the batter and dough recipes. Some baking powders also contain cornstarch. A leavening agent free from cornstarch and egg white may be prepared as follows: 1-1/8 tsp. cream of tartar plus ½ tsp. baking soda. This is equivalent to 1 tsp. of baking powder. This must be mixed as needed.

Wheat-, Milk- and Egg-Free Recipes

SPICE CAKE

Yield: 1 loaf cake
Ingredients

Brown Sugar	1 cup
Water	1¼ cup
Raisins, seedless	1 cup
Citron, cut fine	2 oz.
Fat	1/3 cup
Salt	½ tsp.
Nutmeg	1 tsp.
Cinnamon	1 tsp.
Baking Powder	4 tsp.
Cornmeal, fine	1 cup
Rye Flour	1 cup

Method

1. Boil sugar, water, fruit, fat and salt together. When cool, add to sifted dry ingredients. Mix thoroughly.

2. Bake in a greased loaf pan at 375°F. for about 45 min.

OAT FLOUR NUT MUFFINS

Yield: 6 muffins
Ingredients

Oat Flour	1 cup
Baking Powder	4 tsp.
Sugar	2 tsp.
Salt	¼ tsp.
Water	½ cup
Cottonseed Oil	1 tbsp.
Walnuts, chopped	½ cup

Method

1. Sift dry ingredients together. Add water, oil and nuts. Mix.

2. Fill muffin pans, greased with cottonseed oil, 2/3 full.

3. Bake at 400°F. for about 30 minutes.

FRUIT PUDDING

Yield: 2 servings
Ingredients

Rye Wafers (such as Ry-Krisp)	10
Pineapple Juice	¾ cup
Lemon Juice	2 tsp.
Brown Sugar	2 tbsp.
Cloves	1/8 tsp.
Cinnamon	1/8 tsp.
Nutmeg	1/8 tsp.
Seedless Raisins	¼ cup

Method

1. Roll rye wafers into coarse crumbs or put through coarse blade of food grinder. Mix with other ingredients. Pour into greased dish.

2. Bake at 350°F. for about 1 hour.

3. Serve warm or cold with a sweet fruit sauce or a sugar sauce.

Variations: The pudding may be steamed for 90 min.

OAT PEANUT BUTTER COOKIES

Yield: 1 doz. cookies
Ingredients

Sugar	½ cup
Peanut Butter	1 tbsp.
Cottonseed Oil	2 tsp.
Water	¼ cup
Oat Flour	1½ cups
Baking Powder	2 tsp.

Method

1. Mix sugar, peanut butter and oil. Add water.

2. Add oat flour and baking powder; mix thoroughly.

3. Drop from a teaspoon on cookie sheet greased with cottonseed oil.

4. Press down each cookie with tines of fork. Bake at 400°F. until golden brown.

5. Remove from baking sheet as soon as taken from oven.

RICE PEANUT BUTTER MUFFINS
Yield: 6 muffins
Ingredients

Rice Flour	1 cup
Baking Powder	4 tsp.
Salt	¼ tsp.
Sugar	2 tbsp.
Cottonseed Oil	1 tbsp.
Water	½ cup
Peanut Butter	3 tsp.

Method

1. Sift dry ingredients together. Add oil, water and peanut butter. Mix.

2. Fill muffin pans, greased with cottonseed oil, 2/3 full.

3. Bake at 425°F. for about 20 minutes.

HAWAIIAN MEAT LOAF
Yield: 6 portions
Ingredients

Ground Veal	1 lb.
Ground Cooked Ham, firmly packed	1 cup
Minute Tapioca	2 tbsp.
Salt	1 tsp.
Crushed Pineapple, drained	½ cup
Pineapple Juice	½ cup
Brown Sugar	2 tbsp.

Method

1. Combine meats, tapioca, salt, pineapple and juice. Mix well.

2. Shape into loaf in shallow baking pan; sprinkle brown sugar over top.

3. Bake in moderate oven (350°F.) for about 1 hour.

4. Serve with gravy made from drippings and cornstarch, if desired.

FRUIT TAPIOCA

Yield: 4 to 6 servings

Ingredients

Diced Fruit (canned pineapple, fresh or canned peaches*)	1 cup
Powdered Sugar	2 tbsp.
Fruit Juice	2 cups
Sugar	¼ cup
Salt	¼ tsp.
Minute Tapioca	4 tbsp.
Lemon Juice	½ tsp.

Method

1. Mix fresh fruit with powdered sugar and allow to stand. Heat juice to boiling.

2. Mix sugar, salt and tapioca and add to boiling juice.

3. Boil until clear. Remove from fire and add lemon juice and fruit.

4. Chill and serve with sliced fruit.

*Apricots or red cherries may also be used.

STUFFED PEPPERS

Yield: 4 servings

Ingredients

Rye Wafers (such as Ry-Krisp), crushed	8
Green Peppers, medium sized	4
Fat	½ tbsp.
Ground Beef, lean	½ lb.
Onion, finely cut	¼ cup
Celery, finely cut	¼ cup
Canned Tomatoes, broken, drained	1/3 cup
Salt	¾ tsp.

Method

1. Wash green peppers; slice off tops; remove seeds. Put peppers in pan, cover with boiling water and boil gently 5 minutes. Drain.

2. Melt fat in skillet. Add beef and cook over moderate heat until brown, breaking with fork while cooking. Remove from heat.

3. Add rye wafer crumbs, onion, celery, tomatoes and salt. Mix well.

4. Fill peppers with meat mixture.

5. Stand peppers upright in baking dish. Add hot water to 1-in. depth. Cover and bake about 1 hour at 350°F.

APRICOT AND PINEAPPLE DELIGHT

Yield: 4 servings

Ingredients

Lemon Gelatin	4 tbsp.
Boiling Water	1 cup
Apricot Pulp (dried apricots)	4 tbsp.
Pineapple, diced	4 tbsp.

Method

    1. Dissolve lemon gelatin in boiling water.

    2. Chill until slightly thickened.

    3. Add apricot pulp and diced pineapple. Pour into mold and chill until firm.

    4. Garnish with nuts and cherries.

RYE BREAD

Yield: 2 loaves

Ingredients

Compressed Yeast	1 cake
OR	
Dry Yeast	1 envelope
Water, lukewarm	1-1/3 cups
Sugar	2 tbsp.
Salt	1½ tsp.
Shortening, melted	2 tbsp.
Light Rye Flour	Approx. 5 cups

Method

Crumble compressed yeast or empty envelope of dry yeast into large bowl. Add 1/3 cup of the lukewarm water and 1 teaspoon sugar. Stir and let stand 5 minutes.

Add remaining sugar, salt and shortening. Stir until well mixed. Stir in half the flour and beat until smooth.

Sprinkle about ½ cup of remaining flour on kneading board. Knead until smooth and elastic. Place in greased bowl, cover with a towel and let rise over hot water until double in bulk.

Divide into two parts and shape each on floured board, kneading until mixture can be shaped into a loaf. Place in greased bread pan and let rise until double.

Bake in a moderately hot oven (425°F.) until lightly browned (about 45 min.). Lower temperature to 350°F. and continue baking about 30 minutes more.

ROLLED OATS BISCUITS

Yield: 12 biscuits
Ingredients

Rolled Oats, finely ground	2 cups
Salt	1 tsp.
Baking Powder	3 tsp.
Shortening	3 tbsp.
Water	3/8 to 1/2 cup

Method

   Mix ground rolled oats thoroughly with salt and baking powder. Cut in shortening until mixture is as fine as coarse cornmeal. Stir in enough water to make a stiff dough. Pat out and cut into rounds.

   For a drop biscuit, add more water and drop by tablespoonful on baking sheet.

   Bake in hot oven (450°F.) from 10 to 12 minutes.

SCOTCH FINGERS

Yield: 24 2- by 1-in. sq.
Ingredients

Rolled Oats	1 cup
Salt	¼ tsp.
Baking Powder	1½ tsp.
Sugar	2 tbsp.
Warm Water	2 tbsp.
Molasses	2 tbsp.
Melted Shortening	1 tbsp.

Method

   Mix ground oats, salt, baking powder and sugar. Stir in warm water, molasses and melted shortening; mix well.

   Flour board with ground rolled oats. Roll out to a very thin sheet and cut into narrow strips.

   Bake on a greased pan from 15 to 20 min. in a moderately hot oven (425°F.).

Wheat- and Egg-Free Recipes

ORANGE ICING

Ingredients

Orange Juice	3 tbsp.
Powdered Sugar	1 cup
Egg White, unbeaten	1
Salt	dash
Cream of Tartar	1/8 tsp.
Vanilla	½ tsp.

Method

    1. Bring to boiling point only orange juice and powdered sugar.

    2. Place egg white, cream of tartar and salt in small bowl of mixer. Add hot syrup and immediately beat all ingredients at top speed until the icing is of desired consistency to spread, about 3 or 4 min. Add vanilla while beating.

BROWN BETTY

Yield: 6 servings

Ingredients

Oatmeal, uncooked	1¼ cups
Brown Sugar	1 cup
Salt	½ tsp.
Cinnamon	¾ tsp.
Butter or Margarine, melted	2½ tbsp.
Lemon Juice	2 tsp.
Apples, diced	2 cups
Milk	1½ cups
Cornflakes, crumbled	½ cup

Method

    1. Combine oatmeal, sugar, salt, cinnamon, shortening and lemon juice.

    2. In greased 8- by 8- by 2-in. baking dish, arrange alternate layers of apples and oatmeal mixture, beginning with apples and ending with oatmeal mixture.

    3. Add milk. Cover with crumbled cornflakes.

    4. Bake at 350°F. for about 50 min.

LEMON SHERBET

Yield: 3 servings
Ingredients

Lemon Juice	¼ cup
Sugar	½ cup
Salt	dash
Milk	1 cup
Cream	1/3 cup

Method

1. Combine lemon juice, sugar and salt.

2. Combine milk and cream. Add lemon juice, sugar and salt slowly to milk and cream. Freeze in refrigerator tray.

3. When half frozen, beat until smooth but not melted. Freeze until firm.

MERINGUE COOKIES

Yield: 2 doz.
Ingredients

Rye Wafers (such as Ry-Krisp)	10
OR	
Rice Cereal (rice Chex)	1½ cups
Egg White	1
Brown Sugar	¼ cup
White Sugar	¼ cup
Salt	1/8 tsp.
Vanilla	½ tsp.

Method

1. Roll rye wafers into coarse crumbs. (Leave rice cereal whole.) Set aside.

2. Beat egg white until peaks are formed.

3. Fold in brown sugar a tablespoon at a time.

4. Fold in white sugar, salt and vanilla. Mix until all sugar is combined with egg white.

5. Drop from spoon on greased cookie sheet, spacing 2 in. apart. Bake at 300°F. 12 to 15 minutes, or until outside of cookie is dry and very light brown.

6. Remove from pan at once.

PECAN DROP COOKIES

Yield: 20 cookies

Ingredients

Shortening	¼ cup
Brown Sugar	½ cup
Egg	1
Rye Flour	2 tbsp.
Barley Flour	2 tbsp.
Chopped Pecans	¼ cup
Salt	1/8 tsp.
Maple Flavoring	1/8 tsp.
Soda	1/8 tsp.

Method

1. Cream shortening and sugar. Add egg. Sift dry ingredients together and add to creamed mixture, beating well. Add nuts and flavoring. Drop from teaspoon on greased cookie sheet. Bake at 325°F. for 10 to 12 minutes.

DATE BREAD

Yield: 1 loaf

Ingredients

Cornmeal, uncooked	1 cup
Barley Flour	2 cups
Baking Soda	½ tsp.
Baking Powder	2 tsp.
Salt	1 tsp.
Dates, Raisins, or Prunes, chopped	1 cup
Milk	1¼ cups
Molasses	¼ cup
Shortening, melted	2 tbsp.

Method

1. Sift dry ingredients together. Add fruit. Combine milk, molasses and shortening, and add to the first mixture.

2. Beat well and pour into well greased loaf pan. Let rise for 30 minutes.

3; Bake at 350°F. for about 1 hour and 20 minutes.

APPLE STRUDEL

Yield: 5 servings
Ingredients

Cornflakes or Rice Flakes, slightly crushed	3½ cups
Apples, sliced	2 cups
Granulated or Brown Sugar	½ cup
Cinnamon or Nutmeg	½ tsp.
Butter or Margarine	2 tbsp.

Method

1. Butter baking dish. Arrange crumbs and apples in layers, sprinkle the apples with sugar and spices and dot with butter.

2. Cover casserole dish. Bake at 375°F. for about 40 minutes or until apples are soft.

Note: Sprinkle few drops lemon juice on apples, if not tart.

PINEAPPLE RICE BAVARIAN CREAM

Yield: 5 portions
Ingredients

Plain Gelatin	1½ tsp.
Cold Water	¼ cup
Rice, cooked	½ cup
Sugar	2 tbsp.
Salt	1/8 tsp.
Vanilla	½ tsp.
Pineapple, shredded	½ cup
Whipping Cream	½ cup

Method

1. Soak gelatin in cold water five minutes. Dissolve soaked gelatin over boiling water. Add gelatin to rice, sugar and salt. Mix.

2. Cool mixture. Add pineapple and vanilla. Fold in whipped cream.

3. Pour into individual molds and chill.

SAVORY RICE AND BEEF SUPPER

Yield: 6 cups; 5 servings
Ingredients

Green Pepper, chopped	½ cup
Onion, chopped	½ cup
Butter or Margarine	¼ cup
Ground Beef	1 lb.
Tomatoes, No. 2 can	2¼ cups
Hot Water	1 cup
Minute Rice	1-1/3 cups (5 oz.)
Salt	2 tsp.
Pepper	¼ tsp.

Method

1. Saute green pepper and onion in fat over medium heat until lightly browned; stir occasionally. Add beef and continue cooking 5 min. longer, stirring occasionally. Add tomatoes, water, rice, salt and pepper; mix just to moisten all rice.

2. Cover and simmer slowly 15 minutes.

PLAIN CAKE

Yield: 1 layer cake or 6 cupcakes
Ingredients

Shortening	4 tbsp.
Sugar	½ cup
Milk	½ cup + 1 tbsp.
Barley Flour	1 cup
Baking Powder	3 tsp.
Salt	¼ tsp.
Vanilla	½ tsp.

Method

1. Sift dry ingredients together. Cream shortening, add sugar, mix well.

2. Add liquid, dry ingredients and vanilla.

3. Bake in greased pan 9- by 9- by 2-in. or muffin pans at 375°F. for 25-30 minutes.

Variations: Barley, rye, rice or a combination of these flours may be used.

OVEN-FRIED CHICKEN
Yield: 3 to 4 portions
Ingredients

Frying Chicken, 2½ to 3½ lb.	1
Salad Oil .	1/4-1/3 cup
Salt and Pepper	
Crushed Cornflakes (4 cups before crushing)	1 cup

Method

    1. Cut chicken in serving pieces. Wash and dry well. Brush or dip pieces in oil; drain. Sprinkle each piece with salt and pepper, and roll in crushed cereal flakes.

    2. Arrange in greased shallow baking dish leaving space between pieces.

    3. Cover tightly, and bake in hot oven, 400°F. for 45-60 minutes, or until chicken is tender. Remove cover during last 20 minutes of baking to brown chicken.

PRUNE WHIP
Yield: 5 servings
Ingredients

Gelatin	1½ tsp.
Cold Water	2 tbsp.
Sugar	¼ cup
Prune Juice, hot	¼ cup
Lemon Juice	2 tbsp.
Whipping Cream	½ cup
Prune Puree	½ cup

Method

    1. Soak gelatin in cold water until softened. Dissolve soaked gelatin in hot prune juice to which the sugar has been added.

    2. Partly cool gelatin mixture and add lemon juice. Chill until cold and syrupy.

    3. Whip mixture until fluffy and thick like whipped cream. Fold in cream, whipped only until thick, and continue beating until mixture is stiff enough to hold its shape.

    4. Fold prune puree into gelatin and cream mixture. Turn into molds and chill until firm.

NUTBUTTER COOKIES

Yield: 4 doz.

Ingredients

Rye Wafers (such as Ry-Krisp)	22
Baking Powder	1 tsp.
Shortening	¼ cup
Peanut Butter	½ cup
Sweetened Condensed Milk	
(not evaporated milk)	1 can
Vanilla	1 tsp.

Method

1. Roll rye wafers into coarse crumbs. Stir in baking powder.

2. Melt shortening. Add peanut butter, milk, and vanilla. Mix until completely blended.

3. Add rye wafer crumb mixture to milk mixture. Stir well.

4. Drop from teaspoon on greased pan about 1½ in. apart. Bake at 350°F. for about 12 minutes. Remove from pan at once.

ORANGE BREAD

Yield: 1 loaf

Ingredients

Peel of 2 oranges	
Sugar	½ cup
Water	½ cup
Barley Flour	2 cups
Sugar	½ cup
Salt	½ tsp.
Baking Powder	3 tsp.
Eggs, beaten	2
Orange Juice	½ cup
Shortening, Melted Orange Mixture	3 tbsp.

Method

1. Cover orange peel with water; boil 10 minutes. Drain. Add more water; boil 10 minutes or until tender. Chop peel in food chopper. Add ½ cup water and sugar, cook orange mixture until thick. Sift dry ingredients together.

2. Add beaten eggs, orange juice, melted shortening and orange mixture. Combine well.

3. Pour into well greased bread pan. Bake at 350°F. for 60-70 minutes.

Wheat- and Milk- Free Recipes

BACON-BARLEY PUFFS

Yield: 6 servings
Ingredients

Bacon	6 slices
Pearl Barley, cooked	2 cups
Egg, beaten	1
Salt	¼ tsp.
Pepper	¼ tsp.
Minced Parsley	1 tbsp.

Method

   1. Line muffin pans with strips of bacon.
   2. Combine remaining ingredients; fill greased muffin pans 2/3 full.
   3. Bake at 400°F. for about 30 minutes.

CRUMB CRUST

Yield: 1 8- or 9-in. pie shell
Ingredients

Rice Cereal (such as Rice Chex)	4½ cups
Sugar	¼ cup
Butter or Margarine	1/3 cup

Method

   1. Roll rice cereal into fine crumbs or put through finest blade of food grinder.
   2. Combine crumbs and sugar. Mix thoroughly.
   3. Melt fat. Pour over crumb mixture. Mix until all crumbs are coated with fat. Pack evenly and firmly onto bottom and sides of greased pie pan.
   4. Bake at 300°F. about 10 minutes. Cool before filling. OR, if you prefer, instead of baking crust, refrigerate 1 hour before filling.

CORN AND OAT MUFFINS

Yield: 8 muffins

Ingredients

Cornmeal	¾ cup
Salt	1 tsp.
Baking Powder	3 tsp.
Sugar	3 tbsp.
Rolled Oats, finely ground	1 cup
Water	¾ cup
Melted Shortening	1 tbsp.
Egg, well beaten	1

Method

Mix and sift cornmeal, salt, baking powder and sugar. Add ground oats and mix well. Add water and melted shortening to beaten egg and stir into flour mixture.

Bake in small muffin pan in moderately hot oven (400° F.) about 25 minutes.

SCOTTISH FANCIES

Yield: 1 doz.

Ingredients

Rolled Oats	1 cup
Salt	½ tsp.
Baking Powder	1½ tsp.
Brown Sugar	½ cup
Egg, well beaten	1
Melted Shortening	1 tbsp.

Method

Mix ground rolled oats, salt, baking powder and sugar. Stir in egg and melted shortening; mix well. Drop from teaspoon on well greased baking sheet. Bake in a slow oven (325°F.) until delicately brown. Remove cakes from pan while hot.

Milk- and Egg-Free Recipes

WHITE BREAD

Yield: 2 loaves

Ingredients

Lukewarm Potato Water (water in which potatoes have been cooked)	2 cups
Shortening	2 tbsp.
Sugar	2 tbsp.
Salt	2 tsp.
Yeast	1 cake
Lukewarm Water	2 tbsp.
White Flour	Approx. 6 cups

Method

1. Combine lukewarm potato water, shortening, sugar and salt. Soften yeast in 2 tbsp.water; add to above mixture.

2. Add about 5 or 6 cups white flour, enough to make a stiff dough. Mix thoroughly.

3. Turn on floured board and knead about 10 minutes, until smooth and satiny.

4. Place dough in warm greased bowl, brush surface lightly with melted shortening, cover and let rise 2 hours.

5. Punch dough down thoroughly in bowl, cover and let rise about ½ hour, or until doubled in bulk.

6. Turn out on floured board. Divide in 2 equal parts.

7. Place in 2 greased loaf pans, brush top with melted shortening, cover and let rich dough rise 1 hour.

8. Bake in hot oven (400°F.) for 40-45 minutes.

CHICKEN AND RICE SUPPER

Yield: 6 servings
Ingredients

Minute Rice	2/3 cup
Salt	¼ tsp.
Boiling Water	¾ cup
Chicken Fat	¼ cup
Flour	¼ cup
Salt	1½ tsp.
Pepper	1/8 tsp.
Chicken Broth	2 cups
Cooked Chicken, diced	1/4-1/3 cup
Onion, chopped	2 cups
Lemon Juice	1 tsp.
Parsley, chopped	2 tbsp.

Method

1. Add rice and ¼ tsp. salt to boiling water. Mix only to moisten rice. Cover and remove from heat. Let stand about 15 minutes.

2. Melt chicken fat. Add flour, salt and pepper. Stir until blended.

3. Add chicken broth gradually, stirring constantly.

4. Cook and stir over medium heat til smooth, thick.

5. Add rice, chicken, onion, lemon juice and parsley to sauce, mixing carefully.

6. Heat thoroughly.

BATTER BREAD

Yield: 16 servings
Ingredients

Cornmeal, uncooked	2 cups
Baking Powder	5 tsp.
Salt	1½ tsp.
Rice, cooked	1 cup
Eggs, beaten	2
Shortening, melted	4 tbsp.
Milk	2¼ cups

Method

1. Sift together cornmeal, baking powder and salt. Mix with rice.

2. Combine eggs, shortening and milk. Add this to first mixture. Beat until smooth.

3. Turn mixture into two well-greased 8-in. square pans. Bake at 425°F. 30 minutes.

Wheat-Free Recipes

PLAIN BUTTER CAKE

Yield: 6 portions

Ingredients

Potato Flour	½ cup
Barley Flour	½ cup
Rye Flour	½ cup
Baking Powder	1 tsp.
Butter or Margarine	½ cup
Salt	dash
Sugar, granulated	1 cup
Egg Yolks, beaten	2
Milk	6 tbsp.
Flavoring	1 tsp.
Egg Whites, beaten	2

Method

1. Sift flour with baking powder and salt. Cream shortening and sugar.

2. Add beaten egg yolks and mix until creamy.

3. Alternately add milk and flour mixture. Beat well. Add flavoring.

4. Fold in stiffly beaten egg whites.

5. Pour into 8-in. square greased pan.

6. Bake in oven 350°F. for 25 to 30 minutes.

Variations

1. Cut in half and ice as 2-layer cake.

2. Add 1 square melted chocolate.

3. Add 1 tsp. mixed spices.

4. Add ¼ cup chopped nuts to batter or put on top of cake and omit icing.

REFRIGERATOR PINEAPPLE PIE

Yield: 1 pie

Ingredients

Soft Butter or Margarine	2 tbsp.
Shredded Coconut	1½ cups
Unflavored Gelatin	1 tbsp.
Cold Water	¼ cup
Eggs, separated	3
Crushed Pineapple, undrained	1 cup
Granulated Sugar	¼ cup
Lemon Rind, grated	1 tsp.
Lemon Juice	3 tbsp.
Salt	¼ tsp.
Sugar	6 tbsp.

Method

1. Spread fat evenly on bottom and sides of 9-in. pie pan. Add coconut and spread evenly over fat, pressing down firmly to form pie shell. Bake at 360°F. for 12-15 minutes or until golden brown. Cool.

2. In the meantime, mix gelatin and ¼ cup cold water. In double boiler, mix egg yolks with pineapple, sugar, lemon rind, juice and gelatin mixture.

3. Cook, stirring frequently, for 10-15 minutes or until smooth and thickened.

4. Remove from heat and cool slightly. Beat egg whites and salt until stiff, gradually adding 6 tbsp. sugar.

5. Fold in pineapple mixture. Put in coconut crust. Refrigerate.

SOUR CREAM COOKIES

Yield: 3 doz.
Ingredients

Rye Flour	2/3 cup
Rice Flour	½ cup
Cornstarch	½ cup
Baking Powder	1 tsp.
Salt	¼ tsp.
Butter or Margarine	1/3 cup
Sugar	2/3 cup
Egg, well beaten	1
Thick Sour Cream	1/3 cup
Sugar	1 tbsp.
Cinnamon	¼ tsp.

Method

1. Sift flour, cornstarch, baking powder and salt together. Cream fat, sugar together til light and fluffy. Add beaten egg.

2. Add flour mixture alternately with cream, beginning and ending with flour mixture. Beat until smooth after each addition. Drop by spoon on greased baking sheet.

3. Flatten slightly with bottom of glass which has been dipped in sugar.

4. Mix tablespoon of sugar with cinnamon and sprinkle small amount on top of each cookie. Bake at 357°F. for 15 minutes or until brown.

CORN SOUFFLE

Yield: 3 servings
Ingredients

Butter or Margarine	1 tbsp.
Rice Flour	1 tsp.
Cream	¼ cup
Egg yolk, beaten thick	1
Egg White, beaten stiff	1
Whole Kernel Corn	1/3 cup
Salt and Pepper	dash

Method

1. Melt shortening, add rice flour. Add cream and heat until thickened.

2. Add mixture slowly to egg yolk. Carefully fold in stiffly beaten egg white.

3. Add corn, salt and pepper. Put in ungreased casserole.

4. Bake at 350°F. for 15 minutes and then at 400°F. for about 15 minutes.

DOUGHNUTS

Yield: 12 doughnuts
Ingredients

Eggs, beaten	2
Vanilla	1 tsp.
Sugar	½ cup
Milk	½ cup
Melted Shortening	1½ tbsp.
Rye Flour	2 cups
Baking Powder	3 tsp.
Salt	½ tsp.

Method

1. Beat eggs and vanilla together. Slowly add sugar, beating constantly.

2. Stir in milk and melted shortening. Add sifted dry ingredients. Mix.

3. Roll on a well-floured board to ½-in. thickness. Shape with cutter and deep fry at 380°F. until browned. Drain on unglazed paper.

CREAM PUFFS

Yield: 12
Ingredients

Butter	½ cup
Water	1 cup
Salt	½ tsp.
Wheat Flour*	1 cup
Eggs	4

Method

1. Heat fat, water and salt to boiling point. Add flour all at once to hot liquid, stirring constantly until mixture leaves sides of pan and clings to spoon.

2. Remove from heat. Cool slightly. Add unbeaten eggs one at a time. Beat to a smooth paste after each addition. Drop by spoon onto slightly greased cookie sheet 1½ in. apart. Bake at 410°F. for 10 min., then reduce heat gradually.

*If substitution for wheat flour is desired, see combinations of flours to be used in place of 1 cup wheat flour p. 328. For all flours, except when all rice flour is used, it is best to bake cream puffs at 410°F. for 10 minutes, 350°F. for next 15 or 20 minutes, and finish baking at 300°F. They should generally bake for an hour or slightly less.

RICE AND SALMON PATTIES

Yield: 4 servings
Ingredients

Minute Rice	2/3 cup
Boiling Water	¾ cup
Salmon, drained and flaked (1 lb. can)	2 cups
Mayonnaise	½ cup
Lemon Juice	1 tbsp.
Minced Onion	1 tsp.
Salt	¾ tsp.
Pepper	¼ tsp.
Cornflakes, finely crushed	½ cup

Method

1. Add rice to boiling water in saucepan. Mix just to moisten all rice. Cover and remove from heat. Let stand about 15 minutes.

2. To rice, add salmon, mayonnaise, lemon juice, salt and pepper. Mix well. Let stand 5 minutes. Shape into 8 patties and roll in crushed cereal. Store in refrigerator several hours. Place on greased baking sheet. Bake in hot oven (450° F.) for 15 minutes or until browned. Serve with chili sauce.

VIRGINIA SPOON BREAD

Yield: 6 servings
Ingredients

Milk	3 cups
Cornmeal	½ cup
Eggs, beaten	3
Butter or Margarine	2 tbsp.
Rice, cooked	1 cup
Salt	1¾ tsp.

Method

1. Scald 2½ cups milk, slowly stir in cornmeal mixed with ½ cup cold milk. Cook until moderately thick (about 5 minutes).

2. Remove from heat and add small amount to beaten eggs.

3. Combine eggs, fat, rice and salt with the rest of hot mixture.

4. Turn mixture into a greased baking dish and bake at 325°F. or at 400°F. in a pan of hot water, 45 min. to 1 hour.

WELSH RAREBIT

Yield: 1 serving

Ingredients

Butter or Margarine	1 tbsp.
Rice Flour	2 tsp.
Salt	1/8 tsp.
Milk	¼ cup
Cream	¼ cup
American Cheese, grated	2 tbsp.
Egg, well beaten	1
Paprika (if allowed)	1/8 tsp.

Method

1. Melt shortening, add flour and salt.
2. Slowly add milk and cream; stir until thickened.
3. Add grated cheese. Cook over boiling water until cheese is melted.
4. Stir small amount of hot mixture into beaten egg, then pour back into remaining mixture and cook until smooth.
5. Add paprika, if desired.
6. Serve on toasted rye wafers (such as Ry-Krisp).

OATMEAL COOKIES

Yield: 3 doz. 3-in. cookies

Ingredients

Rye Flour	1 cup
Baking Powder	½ tsp
Salt	½ tsp.
Cinnamon	¼ tsp.
Shortening	½ cup
Cloves	¼ tsp.
Brown Sugar, firmly packed	¾ cup
Egg, well beaten	1
Rolled Oats	¾ cup
Nut meats, chopped	½ cup
Seeded Raisins	½ cup
Sour Milk or Buttermilk	2 tbsp.

Method

Mix flour, soda, salt and spices. Cream shortening, add sugar slowly and cream until fluffy. Stir in well beaten egg, add rolled oats, nutmeats and raisins; mix well. Stir in dry ingredients alternately with sour milk or buttermilk. Drop by teaspoonfuls on greased baking sheet and let stand a few minutes. Flatten dough by stamping with a glass, covered with a damp cloth.

Bake in slow oven (325°F.) from 10 to 15 minutes.

Milk-Free Recipes

BANANA BREAD

Yield: 2 small loaves
Ingredients

Shortening	½ cup
Sugar	1 cup
Eggs	2
Cold Water	½ cup
Bananas	3
Flour	2½ cups
Baking Powder	1 tsp.
Soda	1 tsp.
Salt	¼ tsp.

Method

    1. Cream shortening and sugar. Add eggs and cold water. Mix. Add mashed bananas.

    2. Add sifted dry ingredients. Mix well.

    3. Pour into 2 small greased loaf pans. Bake for about 60 minutes at 350°F.

SPONGE CAKE

Yield: 1 loaf cake
Ingredients

Cake Flour	1 cup
Salt	¼ tsp.
Egg Yolks, beaten	4
Sugar	1 cup
Lemon Juice	4 tsp.
Egg Whites, beaten	4

Method

    1. Sift dry ingredients. Beat egg yolks until thick and lemon-colored. Add sugar gradually, beating constantly. Add lemon juice and mix.

    2. Fold in flour, alternately with stiffly beaten egg whites. Do not beat.

    3. Bake at once in a floured, ungreased loaf pan, about 8- by 4- by 3-in. deep.

    4. Bake at 325°F. for 40-60 minutes.

Egg-Free Recipes

FUDGE CAKE

Yield: 8 servings
Ingredients

Brown Sugar	1 cup
Shortening	2 tbsp.
Flour	1½ cups
Soda	1 tsp.
Baking Powder	1 tsp.
Cocoa	2 tbsp.
Sour Milk	1 cup

Method

1. Cream shortening and sugar. Sift dry ingredients together. Add milk and flour mixture alternately.

2. Pour into greased and floured pans. Bake at 350°F. for 25-30 minutes.

3. Use any desired icing.

GRAHAM-CRACKER BROWNIES

Yield: 16 2-in. squares
Ingredients

Graham Crackers	24
Chocolate Bits	1 6-oz.pkg.
Sweetened Condensed Milk	1 15-oz.can

Method

1. Make graham cracker crumbs by crushing crackers in plastic bag, or between two sheets of wax paper, with rolling pin. Place in bowl.

2. Add chocolate bits and condensed milk. Mix.

3. Place in greased pan 8- by 8- by 1½-in., spreading batter into corners.

4. Bake in moderate oven, 425°F. for 20 to 25 min.

5. Cut into 2-in. squares and remove from pan while still warm.

Note: For chewy brownie, avoid overbaking.

EGGLESS MAYONNAISE

Yield: 1½ cups
Ingredients

Salt	1 tsp.
Paprika	½ tsp.
Sugar	1 tsp.
Dry Mustard	1-1/8 tsp.
Evaporated Milk, undiluted	1¼ cup
Salad Oil	1 cup
Lemon Juice	1 tbsp.
Vinegar	1 tbsp.

Method

1. Ingredients should be cold. While mixing, set the bowl in a pan of ice water.

2. Mix salt, paprika, sugar and dry mustard. Add evaporated milk.

3. Add 1/3 cup of the salad oil, a teaspoon at a time. Beat well after each addition.

4. Combine lemon juice and vinegar. Add a small amount at a time, alternating with remaining salad oil. Beat well after each addition.

5. Store in covered jar in refrigerator.

DATE PUDDING

Yield: 8 servings
Ingredients

Seeded Dates, cut fine	1 lb.
Soda	1 tsp.
Boiling Water	1 cup
Sugar	1 cup
Butter or Margarine	1 tbsp.
Flour	1½ cups
Vanilla	1 tsp.

Method

1. Mix dates, soda and boiling water. Stir well and cool.

2. Mix sugar, shortening and flour. Stir into date mixture. Add vanilla.

3. Pour into well greased baking dish. Bake about 45 minutes at 375°F.

4. Serve with a topping.

Note: This recipe can be doubled and served as a cake.

About the Author

Brother **Herman E. Zaccarelli** is currently Director of Educational Research and Development at Cahners Books in Boston, Massachusetts. His experience covers over 20 years in the foodservice field. He was founder and first director of the International Food Research and Educational Center at North Easton, Massachusetts. He has authored seven books on food service and nutrition. He has written more than 100 articles for food service magazines and journals.

Brother Herman was recently awarded the International Man of Achievement Award by the International Biographical Centre in Cambridge, England, for distinguished service as a humanitarian, social activist, and food service educator. He has served as a consultant on the development of feeding programs for the elderly in various sections of the United States. He attended Cornell University, School of Hotel and Restaurant Administration and completed further studies in food service management at George Washington University, Washington, D.C. He currently serves as Chairman of the Allied Association Committee of the Council of Hotel, Restaurant and Institutional Education, and is a member of the Board of Directors of the Massachusetts Food Service Executives Association. He is a member of the Board of Advisors of the Catholic Golden Age of United Societies of U.S.A.

He is a member of the Congregation of the Holy Cross, and is listed in the 1975 edition of *Who's Who in Religion.*

A noted speaker within the foodservice industry in the United States, he was recently elected to membership in the National Speakers Association.